FASHION
TERMINOLOGY

FASHION TERMINOLOGY

Joane E. Blair
West Valley College

fashion illustrations by

Robert A. Corder
Academy of Art College

Prentice Hall
Englewood Cliffs, New Jersey 07632

Library of Congress Cataloging-in-Publication Data

Blair, Joane E.
    Fashion terminology / Joane E. Blair ; fashion illustrations by
Robert A. Corder.
        p.   cm.
    ISBN 0-13-299355-4
    1. Fashion--Terminology.   I. Corder, Robert A.   II. Title.
TT503.B53   1992
391'.001'4--dc20   91-24200
                                                          CIP

Acquisition editor: *Maureen P. Hull*
Production editor and interior
    design: *Jacqueline A. Martin*
Cover designer: *Bruce Kenselaar*
Cover illustration: *Robert A. Corder*
Prepress buyer: *Ilene Levy*
Manufacturing buyer: *Ed O'Dougherty*
Editorial assistant: *Marianne J. Bernotsky*

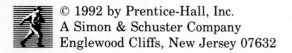
Printed in the United States of America
10 9 8 7 6 5 4 3 2 1

ISBN 0-13-299355-4

Prentice-Hall International (UK) Limited, *London*
Prentice-Hall of Australia Pty. Limited, *Sydney*
Prentice-Hall Canada Inc., *Toronto*
Prentice-Hall Hispanoamericana, S.A., *Mexico*
Prentice-Hall of India Private Limited, *New Delhi*
Prentice-Hall of Japan, Inc., *Tokyo*
Simon & Schuster Asia Pte. Ltd., *Singapore*
Editora Prentice-Hall do Brasil, Ltda., *Rio de Janeiro*

PREFACE

Fashion is part of the history of people in every era. The terminology of fashion is a language of itself. Those who have careers in the fashion industry, from design and manufacturing to retail, need to know the fashion language in order to speak to one another with a knowledge and understanding of the terms. This fashion terminology book presents the words of fashion and their meaning, as well as illustrations of many of the terms by Robert Corder.

Throughout my career in teaching fashion courses and working in the fashion industry, I have found a need for the explanation and illustration of the terminology, as well as information on retail fibers and fabrics and their characteristics. In major categories, the history of fashion terms is explained for the interest and knowledge of the reader. It is hoped that this will be a valuable book for students pursuing a career in fashion, as well as for individuals already established in a fashion career, adding useful knowledge and visual understanding.

ACKNOWLEDGMENTS

My thanks to Robert, for his creativity and enthusiasm for this project. My thanks to the editors of Prentice Hall for their patience and support of this work. Thank you to the following reviewers of the manuscript: Lisa Christman, Auburn University; Louise Hoehn, Virginia Marti College; Selma Rosen, Fashion Institute of Technology; Grace Sonner, College of San Mateo; and Bette E. Tepper, Fashion Institute of Technology. And lastly, my thanks to my husband and family for their encouragement and continual support during the writing of this book.

FASHION
TERMINOLOGY

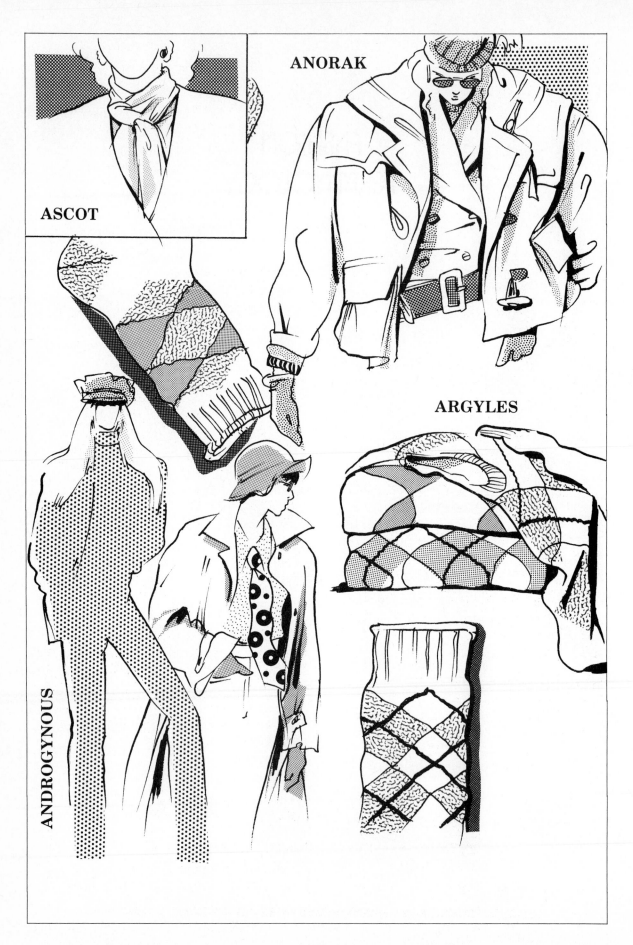

ANORAK

ASCOT

ARGYLES

ANDROGYNOUS

ACCESSORIES Items, other than clothing, to enhance the total "look." Includes jewelry, hair items, hats, cosmetics, glasses, neckwear, belts, hosiery, shoes, handbags, small leather items, billfolds, gloves, sunglasses, and wigs.

ACCORDIAN *see* Pleats

ACETATE Manmade fiber made of chemical compounds of cellulose, cotton linters, or wood chips, with the addition of acetic acid. Developed during World War I for fabric used on the wings of aircrafts. Subsequently produced as fiber made into fabric with properties of drapability, the look of silk, high luster, and some breathability and absorbency. Poor wrinkle recovery and low strength. Usually needs to be dry cleaned.

ACRYLIC A chemically made manmade fiber from acrylonitrile. Early development in Germany, but produced commercially in the United States in 1950 as the first acrylic fiber. Properties include the ability to be spun into high bulk yarns with the look of wool and warmth giving properties. Also lightweight and washable. Acrylic trademarks include "Orlon" by DuPont, "Acrilan" by Monsanto, "Creslan" by American Cyanamid Company, and "Zefran" by Badische. The fibers differ slightly from one manufacturer to another. Acrylic fiber is made into sweaters, knits, socks, sportswear, pile fabrics, and household items.

ADAPTATION Manufacturer's copy of high fashion apparel in less expensive fabrics, to be sold at a lesser price. A copy, a knock-off.

ALENÇON A type of lace.

A-LINE *see* Dresses

ALLIGATOR *see* Leather

ALPACA The strong hair fiber of a domesticated, camel-like animal from the Andes Mountains in South America. Used in making outerwear. Properties include insulation and beauty.

ALPINE JACKET Short, to the waist jacket of Tyrolean origin.

AMETHYST *see* Gemstones

ANDROGYNOUS Used in fashion as a "look" of a female resembling a male. Popularized by movie star Diane Keaton in the 1970's movie *Annie Hall*, and copied as fashion apparel.

ANGORA Long, silky hair fiber of the Angora goat. Also silky fiber of Angora rabbit, with properties of warmth and softness. Rabbit angora sheds easily. Primary use is in sweaters and jackets.

ANKLE STRAP *see* Shoes

ANKLET *see* Socks

ANORAK (ä′ nə räk′) Heavy jacket with hood, from polar areas; parka.

ANTELOPE *see* Leather

APPAREL All categories of clothing worn by women, men, and children.

APPLIQUÉ A method of applying a decorative pattern to the surface of fabric by using cut out pieces of materials and attaching through hand or machine stitches.

APRON A smaller version of apparel used by a woman or man to protect the front of a garment. Also used as a decorative front addition in women's or girl's dresses.

AQUAMARINE *see* Gems

ARAN ISLES The name for a sweater of Irish origin with characteristic cable stitches (braided look). Originated in the Aran Islands, off the southern coast of Ireland.

ARGYLE Diamond shapes in colorful patterns on a solid background. Primarily used in sweaters and socks. Original pattern of the Campbell of Argyle clan.

ASCOT Soft fabric worn around the neck. Forerunner of the tie. Used in today's fashion as a colorful neck accessory. Fabric is knotted with broad ends laid flat on one another. Originally popularized at Ascot, Heath, the famous horse event in Berkshire, England.

ASYMMETRICAL Used in fashion to denote a design line or closure that is off-center. Can be a diagonal or vertical line.

ATTACHÉ CASE A rectangular case to carry documents. Early use of this case by government attachés to carry diplomatic papers. Now used by business professionals. A molded or formed box, made of leather, plastic, or vinyl with top opening and inside pockets for papers, calculators, pens, and other items.

AUSTRIAN CRYSTAL Beads of colored or clear glass, or lead crystal with properties of full light reflection. Used for jewelry.

AVANT-GARDE (à vän gàrd′) A fashion forward or individualistic "look."

B

BABY DOLL *see* Pajamas

BAG Synonymous for handbag.

BAGGIES Fashion pants with added hip/leg fullness.

BAGUETTE *see* Gems

BALLERINA A long, below calf length full skirt. Popular in 1940's and 1950's.

BALLET SHOE A fashion shoe copied from the look of a ballet slipper used by dancers.

BALL FRINGE A braid with tiny balls attached, used to decorate the surface of a garment.

BALLGOWN A long, fashion gown, used for formal occasions.

BALLOON SKIRT *see* Skirt

BALMACAAN *see* Coats

BAND Rectangular fabric used as a collar or cuff. *see* Collar.

BANDANNA A scarf, usually red/white or blue/white checked, used with a Western "look."

BANDEAU (ban dō') 1. A folded horizontal band used as a decorative top of a strapless dress or swimsuit 2. fabric bra top of a 2-piece swimsuit.

BANGLE Round, formed bracelet. Usually worn in groups of two or more.

BARETTE/BARRETTE Small decorative clip to hold hair in place.

BAROQUE Elaborate ornate style of the seventeenth and eighteenth centuries, with much decoration. *see also* Pearls.

BASKET WEAVE Variation of a plain weave. Primarily used for oxford cloth, a shirting fabric.

BATEAU *see* Neckline

BATHING COSTUME/SUIT Innovation of the 1850's. Female version was a complete outfit: dress, bloomers, hat, and shoes. Used to walk into the water. Fabric and design gradually decreased, and in 1922 it became a knitted one-piece, with thigh length shorts, short outer skirt, and sleeveless top. Men's bathing suits of the 1920's were a long, thigh length short and a sleeveless tank top. Men's bathing suits became topless in the 1930's. *see* Swimsuits.

BATISTE Plain weave, soft, fine cotton, or cotton blend fabric.

BATTENBERG A type of lace.

BATTLE JACKET/EISEN-HOWER *see* Jackets

BATWING *see* Sleeves

BEACH PAJAMAS First worn in the 1920's. A woman's one-piece full length culotte jumpsuit. Popular again in the 1970's.

BEADING Use of varieties of beads, sewn onto clothing or accessories for a decorative look. The 1980's reflected much beading on bridal dresses and eveningwear.

BEADS Small shapes of various materials such as glass, pearl, shell, seed, stone, or plastic, with a center hole and strung on narrow cord or leather and worn as a necklace or bracelet.

BEAVER Small water animal pelt used for fur.

BELGIAN A type of lace.

BELL *see* Sleeve; Skirt

BELL-BOTTOM PANTS From nautical look. *see* Pants.

BELT An accessory to secure garment at or near waistline. Early belts of Crete were made of leather and worn tight to emphasize a small waist.

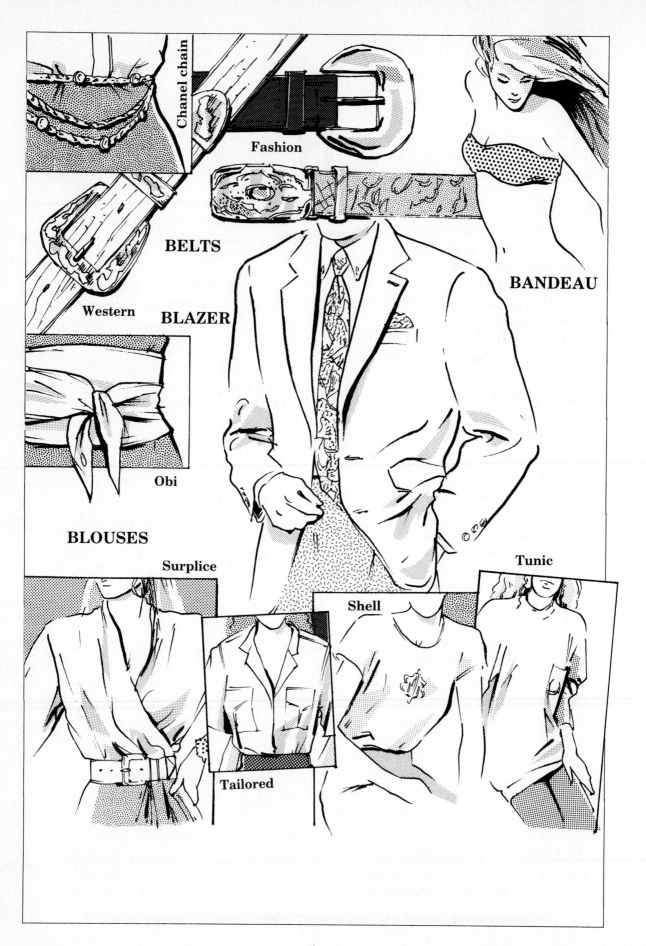

Chanel chain

Fashion

BELTS

Western

BLAZER

BANDEAU

Obi

BLOUSES

Surplice

Tunic

Shell

Tailored

Fashion belts of today may be functional or decorative. Made of fabric, leather, metal, or other materials. Construction may be braided, single layer of material, linked chains (Chanel type), knitted, elastic, contour, Obi style, sash, or cummerbund.

BELT BUCKLE Metal or self fabric device used to fasten belt in place.

BEN FRANKLIN *see* Glasses

BERET (bə rā′) Soft, round cloth cap. Of French origin.

BERMUDA *see* Shorts

BERTHA Large collar, with a cape-like look, often lace trimmed and of contrasting fabric.

BIAS A term used to describe the diagonal cut of fabric. Used in clothing for special effects. Made famous by the French designer Mme. Vionnet in bias cut skirts.

BIB Fabric inset, often of contrasting color or machine tucked, sewn to the front of a garment in neck-chest area. Typically in women's dresses and blouses, and men's tuxedo shirts. Bibs were first worn as extra fabric to protect clothing while eating. Similar use today for infants.

BIKINI *see* Swimsuits; Panties

BILLFOLD Synonymous for "wallet."

BIRD'S EYE Fabric with a small diamond design woven into it.

BISHOP COLLAR/SLEEVE *see* Collars; Sleeves

BLAZER A classic men's and women's jacket. May be single or double breasted, often with metal or non-matching buttons, and worn with contrasting pants or skirts. Men first wore striped or plain blazers with white flannel trousers for summer recreational activities in the early 1900's.

BLEACH Chemical used to whiten fabric or to reduce the intensity of color. Fashion jeans of the 1980's were bleached to reduce the intensity of the indigo color.

BLEED Colors, when applied to fabrics, run or bleed when they become wet. Typical of madras plaid.

BLENDS The use of two or more fibers in the production of yarn. As natural and manmade fibers are blended, the appearance is that of the natural fiber.

BLOCK PRINT Cutting a design into wood or other material, placing into color, and then onto fabric.

BLOOMERS Of Turkish origin. A waist to ankle undergarment, separated into pants and gathered at the ankle. Very popular in the 1920's. Amelia Bloomer introduced the Bloomer Dress in the 1870's. The style failed, but the name remained in reference to women's undergarments.

BLOUSE A garment for the upper part of the body, usually for females. Design details include varieties of collars and sleeve styles. The blouse front is often tucked, gathered, buttoned, pleated, or wrapped for additional design.

Cossack An overblouse with a band collar and sash, of Russian origin.

Middy A slipover blouse with a sailor collar. Of nautical origin.

Overblouse/Tunic A long blouse worn over skirt or pants.

Peasant Typically with a gathered round neckline and gathered puffed sleeves, of ethnic origin.

Shell A short sleeveless, or with cap sleeve blouse, usually without a collar or other design detail.

Tailored Blouse that is shirt-like.

Wrap/Surplice Asymmetrical front with one side overlapping the other.

BLOUSON (bloōs′ än) Jacket or dress that is full at the waist; blouse-like in appearance.

BOA Long scarf of feathers, worn over shoulders with evening gown. Huge feather boas first became popular in the late 1800's.

BOATER Flat top, flat brimmed hat. First introduced for men. A style of hat for women in the 1980's. *see* Hats.

BOAT SHOES *see* Shoes

BOBBY PIN Long U-shaped metal, worn to hold hair in place.

BOBBY SOCKS *see* Socks

BODICE (bäd′ is) The term for the upper part of a dress, from waist to neck.

BODYWEAR Category of clothing used for exercising and dance, consisting of leotard (body suit), tights (leg cover) or unitard (all-in-one—neck to ankle).

BOLERO A short-waist length jacket with curved lower edge, with or without sleeves. Often decorated with braid or other trimmings. Of European origin. *see* Jackets.

BOLO Thin Western type shoelace tie with slide fastener to keep ends in place at neckline.

BOMBER *see* Battle Jacket

BONDING Permanent adhesive used to glue a backing fabric such as tricot, to an outer fabric to give additional stability or warmth.

BONING Plastic strips sewn to garment such as a corset or strapless dress to help keep garment in place.

BONNET A full head covering for infants and young girls to protect from cold or sun. Plastic rain bonnets are a head covering for women to protect the hair from moisture. Easter bonnets of past decades were women's new spring hats. In the 1980's the women's sun hat with wide brim replaced the sun bonnet of the early 1900's.

BOOTEE/BOOTIE Soft foot covering for infants.

BOOTS Foot covering which includes shoe area and extends to ankle or knee. Boots have been in use since 2000 B.C. and have been, through the centuries, both decorative and functional.

Après-ski After ski boot, worn for warmth and fashion.

Courrèges (koo rĕzh′) Short white boot introduced by French designer of same name, popular with the miniskirt of the 1960's. Also called "go-go" boot.

Cowboy/Western A heeled, leather boot for horseback riding, often highly decorated.

Fashion A boot of leather or suede, in fashion colors to coordinate with leather or other apparel.

Hiking Above the ankle boot with inside cushion for comfort and well-made for durability.

Military/Combat Boot made specifically for needs of military.

Riding/jodphur (jäd′ par) Boot for Eastern horseback riding.

Sport Boots made for individualistic sport needs: for example, skating, fishing, skiing, etc.

Utility Boot made specifically for those who work in police, forestry, etc.

BOUCLÉ (boō klā′) Fashion fabric characterized by looped surface.

BOUFFANT (boō fänt′) A full fashion look, as in a skirt with many petticoats or crinolines to achieve fullness. Of French origin.

BOUTIQUE (boō tēk′) A shop/store with limited quantities and styles of merchandise. A specialization of more unusual items. Large department stores of the 1980's enclosed large floor areas of their fashion merchandise to resemble small boutiques.

BOUTONNIÈRE (bōōt″n yer) Flower worn by men in lapel for special occasions.

BOW Rectangular fabric tied with two loops allowing the two tie ends to hang downward. A small tie when worn by men. Varying in size when worn by women.

BOXER Type of shorts copied from the style worn by those in the boxing sport.

BRA From the French word "Brassiere." Undergarment to cover and usually help support a woman's breasts. In the 1920's the breasts were covered with "bandeaus," tight, bust flattening brassieres. The corset of the 1900's was replaced in the 1930's by the "foundation" garment, an all-in-one torso support. By the end of the 1930's, the bra had been detached from the overall foundation into a garment with two cups to cover and support female breasts, with straps over the shoulders and fabric extending around the body with a back closure. The 1960's were characterized by the Feminist Movement and "burn the bra" was a common statement. Thus many women became braless. John Kloss, the designer, is credited with the return of the bra in the 1970's, by designing bras using feminine colors, laces, and other adornment. Bra fronts are of various styles, with full breast cover, demi or partial cover, and plunge, with a deep front opening. Soft bra cups or full support cups are built in to many women's swim suits.

Padded Bra Additional fiberfill or other fabric is added to the cups to give more fullness to the wearer.

Soft Cup Powerstretch fabric with cup shaping, and front, or back closure.

Sport Bra Special for active sports, with a tank type front, V or T back for additional comfort when participating in the sport.

Strapless Underwire type bra, lace or fabric cups, and no shoulder straps. Can also be made in a long line to the waist. Otherwise known as a "Merry Widow" which controls the body fullness to the waist.

Underwire A bra with a curved wire under the breasts for added support and to keep the breasts in place. The cups are of stretch fabric and/or lace.

BRACELET Jewelry that circles the wrists, ankle, or upper arm. The origin of bracelets is noted in early Etruscan civilization and is in continual use until present day. Today's bracelets are made of fine jewelry, like metals and gemstones, as well as costume jewelry made of plastics, metals, woods, leathers, beads, etc.

Ankle Bracelet Worn around ankle; from earliest times. Some use currently, as in I.D. bracelet or chain type ankle bracelet.

Bangle Bracelets of defined form, usually round, worn many at a time and making a jangle noise when arm is moved.

Chain Narrow metal bracelets, often woven or braided.

Charm Use of a metal chain of gold or silver from which metal items are hung, such as grandchildren disks, personal event disks, special memory disks, zodiac signs, or coins.

Cuff Wide bracelet that fits the arm, but does not completely encircle. Has opening for putting on and removing.

I.D. Identification bracelet, of metal, with name of wearer engraved. Now

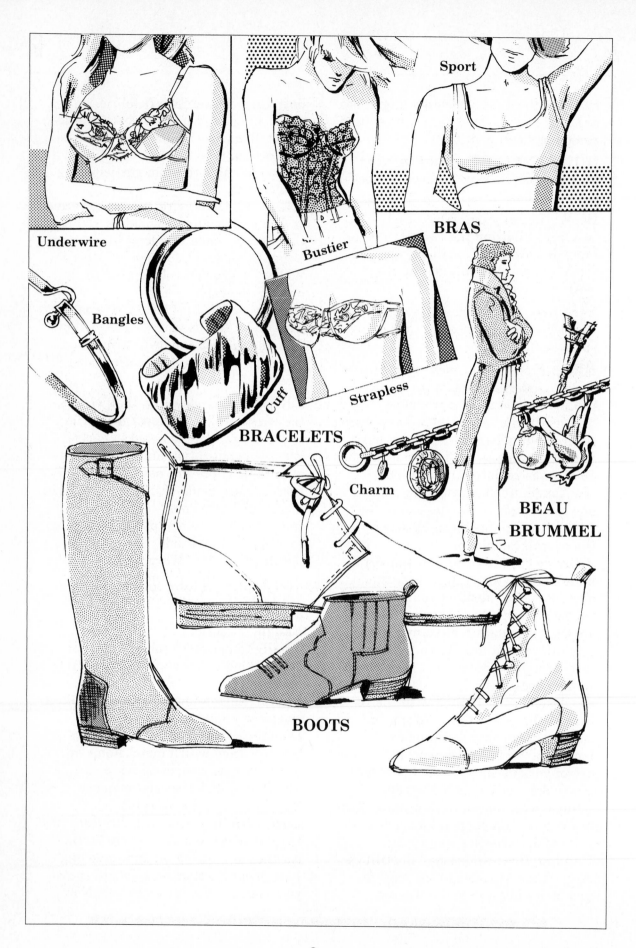

Sport

BRAS

Underwire

Bustier

Bangles

Cuff

Strapless

BRACELETS

Charm

BEAU
BRUMMEL

BOOTS

worn with medical information about the wearer in case of an emergency situation. Also used as "love" bracelets with names of male and female engraved on bracelet.

Tennis Current name given to a narrow metal bracelet studded with diamonds or diamond-like stones.

Watch Bracelet with watch face(s) on it. In the 1980's, the use of many watch faces on one bracelet was fashionable.

BRACES Synonymous for suspenders. Name of British origin.

BRAID 1. Woven fabric used as a trim. Braids are generally narrow and of contrasting colors and used for design effect. 2. Used to denote plaits of hair woven into a braid hairstyle.

Middy A flat, narrow contrasting braid used for nautical effect.

Military Usually flat, gold-type braid, used on uniforms or military type apparel.

Rickrack Type of zigzagged, narrow fabric, used for braid effect.

Soutache (soo tash') Flat, narrow braid, usually made into elaborate floral or other designs and sewn to apparel and accessories for design effect.

BRASSIERE *see* Bra

BREECHES Early term for men's trousers. *see* Jodphurs.

BRETON A type of lace. *see also* Hats.

BRIDAL All clothing and accessories worn by a bride for a wedding.

BRIDGE Items of fashion merchandise that are designed and priced between very high and budget/moderate. Bridge jewelry: use of semi-precious gemstones and metals with the look of fine jewelry, of lesser quality and price.

Many current designers are doing a line of clothing, lesser in price than their top line and termed their "bridge" line.

BRIEFS Men's form-fitting, knitted underwear, usually with elastic waist. Also used as a term for women's underwear. *see* Panties.

BRIM Outer extended rim of a hat. May extend straight, curved, or any style the designer chooses.

BROADCLOTH Originally a fine wool fabric with slight napping. Now a cotton or manmade blend, major use for shirting.

BROCADE Elegant patterned fabric achieved by weaving on jacquard loom. Design on face of fabric is raised, with floats on the back. Major fashion use is in eveningwear.

BROGUE *see* Oxford shoe

BROOCH *see* Pins

BRUMMELL, GEORGE BRYAN (BEAU) An English "dandy" wearing a high fashion look in the early 1800's, and widely copied. Typified by ankle length trousers, fitted knee length jacket (frock coat), starched collar, and elegantly tied cravat.

BRUSSELS A type of lace.

BUBBLE Large, bouffant hair style of 1950's. Also a skirt silhouette. *see* Dress.

BUCKLE A clasp to fasten belts and other closures. Usually of metal, self fabric, wood, or plastic, with metal bar or tongue to insert in opposing hole to secure.

BUCKSKIN *see* Leathers

BULKY Usually referring to large stitched knit apparel, or a large silhouette.

BURBERRY Trademark for an English designed raincoat, commonly used word for "rain coat."

BURLAP Fabric made of plain, loosely woven jute. Some use in fashion handbags and totes.

BURNOOSE/BURNOUS (bar noos') Very full coat, cape. A hooded wrap with attached tassles.

BUSH Hat, jacket, or pants with "Safari" look.

BUSTIER (bust i ày) Strapless, corsetlike garment. Originally worn under a dress. Made famous as outerwear by a female singer of the 1980's.

BUSTLE (bus' 'l) Fullness added to women's skirts, either at sides, or back, through the use of metal projections, horse hair, or other padding or fabric.

BUTCHER CLOTH Fabric usually of linen or rayon, with slubs for texture effect.

BUTTONHOLE Opening for button. May be made of self fabric, contrasting fabric or thread to finish off open cut area. Two variations: 1. Machine made with visible stitches. 2. Fabric bound edges.

BUTTONS Plain or decorative fastener to put through a buttonhole or fabric loop. Typical kinds of buttons: shirt buttons with two or four exposed holes; covered button of self fabric or leather; metal or crested-metal button; pearl or pearl-like round button, gem, gemlike, or crystal buttons, wood, plastic, ceramic, hand painted, or other designed buttons.

C

CABRETTA *see* Leather

CAFTAN Of Middle Eastern origin. *see* Dresses.

CALFSKIN *see* Leather

CALICO Cotton or cotton blend fabric printed with small flower designs. Named for fabric first imported from Calicut, India. Inexpensive fabric. Early use by American females for "prairie" dresses.

CAMEL'S HAIR Fine hair from the two-humped Bactrian camel native to Asia. Obtained from hair shed by the camel and then woven into soft, fine, luxurious, but not durable, fabric. Camel's hair provides excellent warmth without weight and is used in its natural color of light brown or tan. Used for men's and women's coats, blazers, and suits.

CAMEO A broach-type of jewelry, distinguished by the carving of the face, neck and shoulders of a woman, in a raised design on onyx, agate, or shell. This material has layers of different hues; the raised design is of one color and the background of another.

CAMISOLE A decorative short lingerie top, fitting over bust, ending at waist. Early use was to cover corset top.

CANVAS Close woven coarse fabric of hard twisted yarn of various weights. Considered a strong, durable, utility fabric. Some use in fashion as espadrille tops and summer handbags and totes.

CAP 1. Head covering that firmly fits the head. Varieties include visor-type front, as in baseball and other sport caps, short billed visor, as in Greek and Irish, Dutchboy or men's sport caps, and Touring, men's early automobile cap. Some caps are knitted and fit to the head, as in a ski or child's cap, for cold weather. The Deerstalker cap has visors on both the front and back, with ear flaps, also called the Sherlock Holmes. The bathing cap of rubber or other stretch fabric, covers hair while swimming. 2. *see* Sleeves

CAPE A circle or partial circle of fabric that covers shoulders, and range from short to ankle length. Used as outerwear for warmth. Long capes may have side openings for arms. Also may be a decorative design detail added to female or children's clothing. When short, called "Capelet."

CAPRI *see* Pants

CARAT Designated weight for gemstones. Carats (pieces) of gemstones are divided into units called "points." One carat equals 200 milligrams.

CAR COAT *see* Coats

CARDIGAN Front opening knitted garment named after Earl Cardigan of the British Army in the 1700's who made the style famous. *see also* Sweaters.

CARDING Textile manufacturing process of straightening and aligning fibers, taking out shorter fibers to make ready for yarn spinning process. Finished carded fibers are called "sliver."

CARGO *see* Pockets

CARNELIAN *see* Gems

CARPET BAG *see* Handbag

CASCADE 1. A waterfall design effect achieved by use of bias cut ruffles attached vertically or diagonally to the front of a garment or the use of gathered lace for the same effect. 2. A

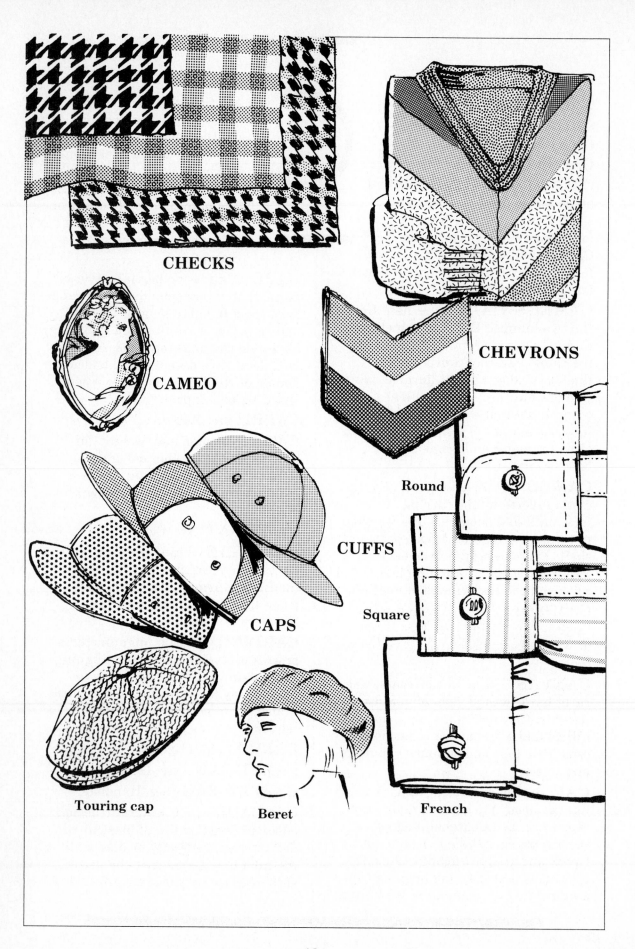

CHECKS

CHEVRONS

CAMEO

Round

CUFFS

Square

CAPS

Touring cap

Beret

French

waterfall design hair style of curls that fall from top of head to back of neck.

CASHMERE Very soft hair of the Cashmere goat. Used in making fine, luxurious knitted apparel such as sweaters and sweater dresses. Mohair has a high luster and is woven for men's and women's suiting. Also used for household fabrics. The cost of mohair is higher than wool. From Kashmir in India.

CASHMERE SHAWL Court shawls of woven hair of the Cashmere goat, beautifully embroidered with colored and/or gold and silver threads.

CASUALWEAR Synonymous with sportswear. Informal clothes worn for comfort and nonformal occasions.

CAT'S EYE *see* Gems

CAT SUIT Stretch, sculptured to the body jumpsuit, originally worn by Diana Rigg on *The Avengers* television series in the 1960's.

CELLULOSE/CELLULOSIC FIBER The use of some plants as a source for fibers, for example, the cotton plant and the flax plant are major natural fiber sources for cotton and linen. Cotton linters or wood pulp, when manufactured, are the basis for rayon and acetate. Other cellulose fibers are ramie, jute, and hemp.

CERISE A brilliant red. Of French origin; means "cherry."

CERULEAN A pale blue-green color.

CHAIN 1. Series of links or rings, usually of metal, connected and fitted into one another. May be of gold, silver, or a base metal material. Made into necklaces or bracelets for arm or leg. In larger form, as chain belts. 2. An embroidery stitch of interlocking loops.

CHALLIS (shal' ē) Lightweight fine fabric, often distinguished by a dark background and a small printed flower design. Soft, drapable fabric of cotton, silk, wool, rayon, or fiber blends.

CHAMBRAY (sham' brā) Plain weave, medium weight fabric of colored warp yarn and white filling yarn. Typically a muted blue color. Used for shirts, sportswear, and the "Western" look.

CHAMOIS (sham' ē) From sheepskin. A sueded finish, soft leather, used for shirting, dresses, jackets. Of French origin.

CHANTILLY A type of lace.

CHAPEAU (sha pō') Older terminology for "hat." Of French origin.

CHAPS 1. Term for leather leggings worn by horserider to protect pants. 2. Ralph Lauren registered trademark.

CHARM Small, decorative object or memento such as a zodiac sign, heart, or other, worn on a chain bracelet or necklace.

CHARMEUSE (shär' müs) A lightweight silk or silklike fabric used for blouses or dresses. Of French origin.

CHARTREUSE (shär trooz') A green/yellow color.

CHECK A square design, usually woven into fabric, but may be printed. Design squares of alternating colors, usually one square is white.
Buffalo Very large checks.
Even As in a checkerboard.
Gingham Small checks of color that alternate with white checks.
Houndstooth A pointed, uneven check, using twill weave to achieve effect.

Windowpane Narrow horizontal and vertical bars, more widely spaced, to give windowpane effect.

CHEMISE *see* Dress

CHENILLE Also called "candle-wick." Fuzzy, faced fabric with cotton warp and pile filling. A fuzzy "caterpillar" appearance. Of French origin.

CHEONGSAM (shong sam) Female silk chemise with skirt side slits and mandarin collar. Often embroidered for added beauty. Of Chinese origin.

CHEVRON A 'V' design created by woven contrasting colored V design or printed V design. Designers often create a chevron design by cutting a stripe on the bias.

CHIC (shēk) A word to describe someone with style and elegance in co-ordinated apparel, accessories, hair styling, and facial cosmetics. Of French origin.

CHIFFON A very sheer fabric of fine, hard twisted yarns of silk, polyester, or other fibers. May be solid color or printed designs.

CHIGNON (shēn′ yän) A knot or roll of hair, real or fake, worn at top of head or nape of neck. Of French origin.

CHINA GRASS From plant fiber called ramie. Of Chinese origination, now grown in other parts of the world. Finished fabric resembles and has the characteristics of linen. *see* Ramie.

CHINA SILK Fine, soft silk fabric, usually used as a lining for a silk or wool garment.

CHINCHILLA *see* Furs

CHINESE KNOT Ornamental knot used as a button, with accompanying loop for a decorative closure.

CHINO (chē′ nō) Firmly woven plain or twill weave cotton or cotton blend. Yellow-tan color. Major use as summerwear pants or shorts for men.

CHINTZ Semi-glazed printed cotton.

CHOKER Term used for necklaces that fit at base and upwards of neck. May be one or several strands.

CIRÉ (sə rā′) Textile term to describe a shiny or wet look to finished fabric.

CIVET Fluid secreted by the civet cat (of Africa and Asia) used in the manufacturing of fragrances for a strong, musk odor.

CLAMDIGGERS *see* Pants

CLASSIC Styles or designs that remain in use over a long period. Fashion that has been accepted for an extended period of time and/or has returned to the fashion cycle periodically. Examples include: shirtwaist dresses, pumps, blazers, trenchcoats, cardigans.

CLEAVAGE Partial exposure of a woman's breasts through wearing low necked apparel.

CLIP Jewelry such as earrings or brooches that are attached with a clip or spring fastener.

CLOCHE (klōsh) Female fitted hat of the 1920's.

CLOISONNÉ (kloi′ zə nā′) Use of decorative colored enamel for patterns on jewelry.

CLOSURES/CLOSINGS Method of fastening apparel or accessory openings.

Button The use of an object with holes for thread, sewn to material and then put through a buttonhole or loop to close.

D-Ring A double ring through which fabric or other material is threaded and overlapped to firmly close.

Frog A decorative closure using a Chinese button/ball and closed with a loop of cording. Also called "Chinese knot."

Gripper/Snap The use of metal fasteners of various sizes, with one protruding center that fits into the hole of the other metal side to close. Larger sizes are usually referred to as grippers. Commonly used in infant clothing and outerwear.

Hook/Eye The use of a metal hook, attached to one side of the opening and fitting around the metal or thread bar on the other side of the opening.

Laced/Tie The use of cord, string, lace, or narrow leather strips to thread through holes and then tied in crisscross fashion to close. Most common use in shoes.

Loop A length of narrow fabric or cording folded over and secured at ends, forming an opening that secures a button closing.

Sash/Tie The use of rectangular fabric to wrap around area to close. Usually secured by a knot. Commonly used to close a wraparound garment such as a skirt, coat, or robe.

Toggle Rectangular object of wood or plastic, used as a button for a closure.

Velcro A woven nylon tape of tiny, interlocking loops that fasten by placing one side of the tape onto the other. First used in space vehicles. Astronauts applied this to the bottoms of their boots to enable them to be attached to one place while in a no gravity atmosphere. A popular closure with much use in childrenswear, shoes, clothing for the elderly, disabled, as well as the fully abled.

Zipper A closure apparatus using "teeth" to interlock and close an opening. Formerly of metal, now of metal or a light weight nylon. First used as apparel closures by Molyneux in the 1930's to close his famous tube jacket.

CLOTH Synonymous for fabric.

CLOTHES Synonymous for apparel.

CLUNY A type of lace.

CLUTCH *see* Handbag

COAT Outerwear apparel, worn for warmth. Of various lengths, designs, silhouettes, and details. The Alba was first worn as an outer wrap in 1000 A.D. The Cotehardie, a significant clothing innovation of early 1100's, was the first true coat. The women's Cotehardie had a fitted top and long gored/flared skirt, with inset sleeves. The men's were similar in style but thigh length. Both were fastened with buttons. Men's coats retained this general style, with additions of collars and lapels.

The coat gradually became long, even ankle length. Women wore capes or mantles with hoods in the eleventh and twelfth centuries, graduating to full length ornamental wraps, often sleeveless and then to full capes. During the elegance of the French Louis kings, women wore variations of the overcloke: wraps, capes, and short jackets over their decorative dress.

The coats of the late 1800's and early 1900's followed the full figured dress forms of that era, with huge dolman sleeves. Evening wraps of the 1920's were as flamboyant as the period. Molyneux created a bulky, full-fronted day coat in the 1930's with large collars, lapels, and sleeves, generally midcalf length. By the 1940's a general stability in style was obtained. Variations in general use today are fitted, straight or full (swing back) silhouette, buttoned or wrapped, with varying hem lengths and design details, and include:

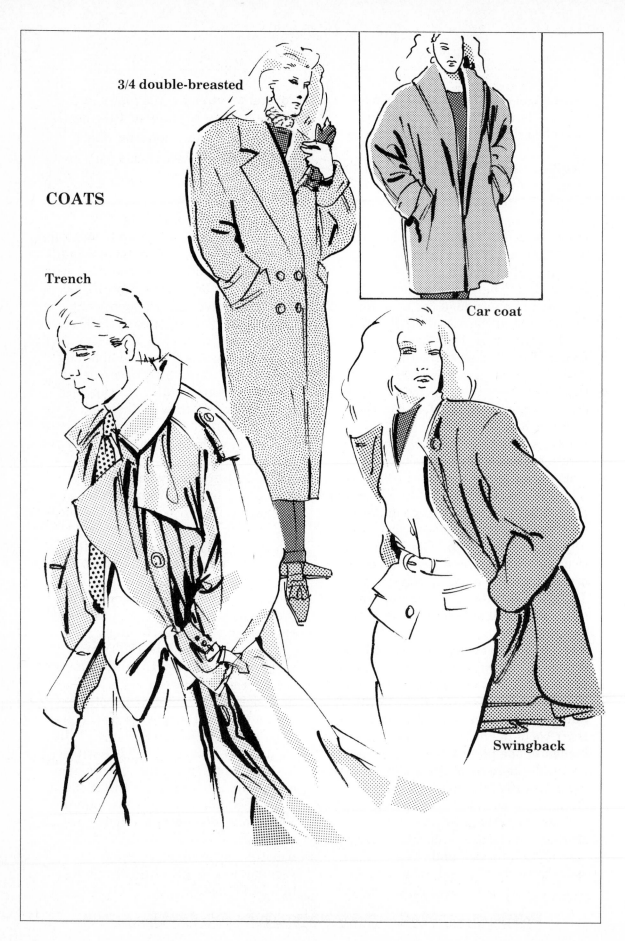

3/4 double-breasted

COATS

Trench

Car coat

Swingback

16

All-weather Typically a raincoat with water repellant properties, and a zip in/out lining for additional warmth.

Car/Pea/Stadium Hip/thigh length coat, originally of nautical origin. Single- or double-breasted. More casual in appearance.

Chesterfield Single- or double-breasted, somewhat fitted coat, characterized by a black velvet or velveteen collar. Introduced in England in the 1860's, originally with a fur collar. Named for the Earl of Chesterfield.

Cocoon Wrap-type coat with narrow silhouette, dolman sleeves. Extends to center front with rounded neck and center front hem.

Cutaway Originated in the 1840's as a man's frock coat. A fitted, waist length front, and long back tails. Now a formal/tuxedo-type coat for men for special occasions.

Double-breasted Coat with overlapping front and a double line of buttons to close front.

Duster A loose, unfitted, lightweight coat of various fabrics such as silk, linen, cotton, or blends of fibers.

Overcoat A man's coat, of various styles, worn as outerwear.

Polo A classic styled, notched collar wrap coat and fabric sash/belt.

Princess Woman's coat of the princess line, with long, fitted vertical panels. Single- or double-breasted.

Reefer A classic-styled, semi-fitted coat, usually single-breasted with larger lapels.

Single-breasted Coat with a single line of buttons to close the front.

Tent/Swingback Woman's coat with considerable lower flare or fullness. The swingback has additional back fullness/flare.

Topcoat Synonymous for overcoat, often more fashion forward.

Trenchcoat Classic-styled raincoat adapted from World World I military coat, with raglan sleeves, epaulets, belted, with a military look.

COBALT BLUE Intense, medium blue color.

COCHINEAL (kӓch′ə nēl′) Bright red color dye made from the dried bodies of a certain female insect found in Mexico.

COIFFURE (kwä fyoor′) A hairstyle; a way to "dress" the hair in a fashionable style. Of French origin.

COIR Fiber derived from the husk of coconut. Used for rope or mats.

COLLAR Decorative piece, detachable or permanently attached to neckline of apparel.

Band Narrow, rectangular collar that is attached at the neckline and extends upward. Sometimes referred to as a stand-up-collar.

Bertha A wide, shoulder covering collar having a V-opening at the center front.

Bishop Extra large collar, rounded in front.

Bow Fabric attached to neckline of garment with ends extending and tied in the form of a bow to close.

Buttondown Classic, shirt collar with collar points buttoned to shirt front.

Convertible A classic shirt collar, usually in more casual design, to be worn buttoned with a tie, or unbuttoned and casual.

Cowl A large drape, sewn to bodice of garment, that lays in folds at the neckline.

Mandarin/Chinese/Oriental A banded collar noted by a center front separation.

Middy/Sailor From nautical. A long square back and tie front collar. Can also be attached in reverse. Often with

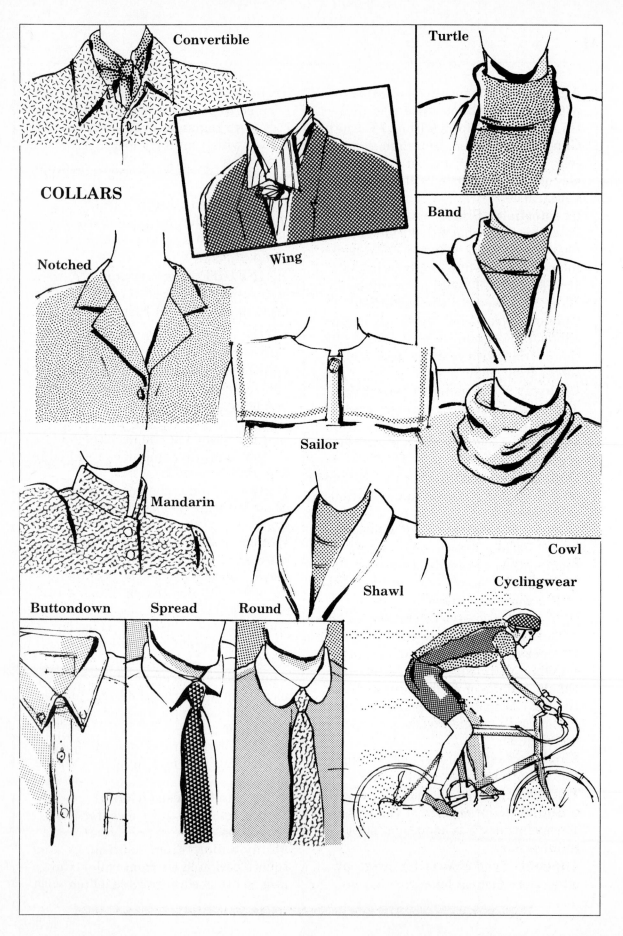

Convertible

Turtle

COLLARS

Wing

Band

Notched

Sailor

Cowl

Mandarin

Shawl

Cyclingwear

Buttondown   Spread   Round

middy braid sewn on for a decorative edging.

Peter Pan Two round-edged, flat collars, separated at center front.

Pierrot 1. Small, rounded double collar, often lace trimmed. Originated in the 1850's. 2. A short, fitted female jacket with ruffled peplum in back, from the 1700's.

Puritan/Pilgrim From early Pilgrim apparel. Large, rounded collar ending in center front points.

Shawl Collar and lapel combined in a single, folded front opening.

Shirt Classic, turned down shirt collar ending in points near center front.

Spread Shirt collar with collar points spread farther apart than classic shirt collar.

Turtle A high, banded collar that fits the neck and rolls back on itself.

Wing Tip/Tuxedo Narrow band collar at back and sides, and front-pointed tips folded down.

COLLECTION Term used to describe a designer or manufacturer's new apparel designs for the season. *see* Line.

COMB A toothed instrument used to untangle or arrange hair. Decorated combs have been used since early Etruscan days to hold hair in place and used for adornment.

COMBING An additional step in the production of yarns, after carding, to further parallel and reduce the number of short fibers. The process is more expensive, but the yarn is of a finer quality. When used with cotton fiber, the result is "combed" cotton.

COMPACT A decorative cosmetic container, with mirror on one side and often containing a blush or other cosmetic product.

COORDINATES Two, three, or more separates (skirt, pants, blouse, sweater) of matching or coordinating fabric and color to form a complete, finished "look."

CORAL *see* Semiprecious gems

CORDING Narrow, tubular fabric with rope or cordlike insert. When narrow, used as a decorative trim on apparel. A fuller cording is also used as a tie belt.

CORDOVAN *see* Leather

CORDUROY A soft, full pile weave fabric with a lengthwise rib effect called wales. Width of wales is from narrow, pin wales, to very wide wales. This fabric is widely used in sportswear for pants, jackets, vests, and childrenswear. Of French origin.

CORE YARN Textile term for a center yarn/fiber, wrapped with another yarn/fiber. Widely used with a Spandex core, wrapped with nylon or cotton.

CORNFLOWER BLUE Color of blue from flower of same name.

CORNROWS Hairstyle of many very narrow rows of braids.

CORSET Woman's one-piece undergarment covering breasts to thighs and holding the body rigid with metal, or whalebone inserts. Originally laced tightly to give the body a narrow, small waist silhouette. Used since the 1700's, but widely used in late 1800's to early 1900's. Found by doctors to be damaging to the body and eventually discarded. Brought back in the 1930's and 1940's lighter weight and less restrictive. Some use today as an all-in-one bra and lower body control undergarment.

COSTUME JEWELRY *see* Jewelry

COTTON Fiber taken from boll or seed pod of cotton plant. Most widely used fiber in the world. Length of the fiber varies from $\frac{3}{8}''$ to some of the finest cotton—Sea Island, Egyptian or pima cotton, which is $1\frac{1}{2}$ to 2 inches in length. Major advantage of this fiber is absorbency and comfort. Cotton is medium strong, affected by mildew, may shrink, and tends to wrinkle.

COTY AWARDS American fashion critics designer awards.

COUNTER Inner reinforcement covering inner heel area of shoe and giving additional form.

COUTURE (kōō toor′) French term meaning *fashion*, and the business of a couturier designer. *Haute couture* is a term for high fashion, meaning original designs from well-known fashion designers.

COUTURE HOUSE The building in which designers work. If well-known, it is named for the designer, for example, "House of Dior."

COUTURIER (kōō tü rya′) Male fashion designer.

COUTURIERE (kōō tü ryēr′) Female fashion designer.

COVERALLS A one-piece worksuit/jumpsuit, usually of heavy-duty and washable fabric.

COVERT CLOTH Twill weave, usually wool, menswear fabric.

COWL *see* Necklines

CRAVAT In the seventeenth century, this began as bands of fabric encircling a man's neck and used as a fashion accessory. In the present century, a type of necktie or scarf worn as a necktie. A tie to accompany a tuxedo.

CREAM A yellow-white color of cream from milk.

CREPE Fabric with a crinkled pebbly appearance, made of yarns with exceptional high twist.

CREPE BACK SATIN Fabric of satin weave with crepe twist filling. Results in one side having a shiny satin appearance and one side having a dull crepe appearance. Either side may be used as the face fabric.

CREPE de CHINE (krāp′ də shēn′) Soft, lightweight fabric with a crinkled effect. Of French origin.

CRESTS Small, ornamental design placed on apparel to indicate some type of royalty or membership in a specific group. Used in fashion to decorate apparel.

CREW NECK *see* Neckline

CRINOLINE Cotton fabric, highly sized, used for stiffening. Former use, stiffened horsehair underskirts to give fullness to the outer skirt.

CROCHET (krō shā′) To create decorative fabric by hand. Making a series of interlocking loops by the use of a crochet hook and yarn. A way of copying the look of lace.

CROCKING Loss of color in fabric when fabric pieces rub together through friction or wear.

CROPPED Term that describes a shortened garment, such as a pant leg or jacket length.

CROTCH The area of a garment/body where two legs meet the torso.

CROWN/TIARA 1. Circular head ornament of precious stones and metals, to denote royalty. 2. The top part of the head and the hat.

CRYSTAL *see* Gems

CUBIC ZIRCONIA *see* Gems

CUE/QUEUE In fashion, a hanging braid of hair in back of head, or a hanging ringlet of hair. A pigtail.

CUFF A separate, fitted band of fabric to finish the lower edge of a sleeve.

Band Rectangular cuff without a separate opening.

Detachable Cuff that can be attached with buttons, snaps, or zipper and removed for cleaning.

French Double cuff that turns back, usually fastened with ornamental cuff links.

Knit A rib knit cuff that expands and returns to shape after hand is placed through.

Single Rectangular cuff with button opening.

CUFFED/CUFFS Term to describe the turn back, bandlike appearance at the lower edge of pants or sleeves.

CULMINATION The stage of the fashion cycle when a fashion is most popular. It is mass-produced at all price points and is purchased and worn by the most people.

CULOTTES *see* Pants

CUMMERBUND Wide, often pleated, sash of fabric, or fabric insert, worn at the waist/rib area of body. Fashion accessory for men's formalwear. Since the 1960's, tuxedos with contrasting, colored, or pleated cummerbunds have been in fashion.

CUSTOM-MADE One-of-a-kind garment, made to client's measurements and specifications.

CUTOUTS Term to describe holes of various shapes/designs, cut in clothing, shoes, swimwear, and other fashion items.

CYCLINGWEAR Apparel worn specifically for bicycle riders. Thigh length, fitted pants with padded crotch for added comfort and coordinated top.

D

DAMASK Fabric made by woven Jacquard technique. Often uses a satin weave for the pattern and a plain or twill weave for the background. White linen damask has long been used for tablecoths, and also in fashion as suiting fabric. Damasks are reversible. May also be of cotton or fiber blends.

DECLINE A decrease in consumer demand for a certain fashion. Individuals continue to wear the fashion, but sales are falling. Fashions in the Decline stage go down much faster, generally, than fashions beginning to Rise.

DÉCOLLETÉ (dā käl′ ə tā′) Word for low, breast-revealing neckline. Of French origin.

DEMI Literally meaning "half." In fashion, as applied to bras, boots, and sleeves, means less than the full size.

DENIM Durable, twill weave fabric of colored warp (lengthwise) yarn and white filling yarn. Typical denim is indigo blue, of cotton or cotton blend fibers. A popular fashion use is for jeans, jackets, and skirts. Denim variations may be in other colors, a faded look, stone wash-distressed look, acid wash distress, and others.

DESIGN To create, sketch, or otherwise invent a new artistic work.

DESIGNER In fashion, the designation for one who has created a new design for fabric, apparel, or accessories. Haute couture designers are known by their names. Designers for manufacturers are not generally known by name, just the product label is known.

DIAMOND *see* Gemstones

DICKEY A false shirt/blouse front, consisting of collar and a short front.

Usually worn under sweaters for a layered look. Could also be a knitted sweater dickey, worn under a blouse or shirt, for same effect.

DIMENSIONAL STABILITY The ability of fibers/fabrics to retain their original shape. Knitted garments, because of their greater stretchability, are more likely to lose shape than woven garments that have greater stability.

DIMITY Sheer fabric of cotton, often with lengthwise cord effect. A plain weave with lengthwise rib variation.

DIRNDL A skirt which is fully gathered at the waistline. Usually attached to a waistband, but may be sewn to a bodice to form a dress. From ethnic origin: Tyrolean, Austrian, Bavarian.

DISPLAY In fashion, the visual presentation of apparel and accessories through use of mannequins or other props. Interior store display and window display.

DOESKIN 1. *see* Leather. 2. Fabrics with sueded (heavy napped) finish, used for apparel.

DOLMAN *see* Sleeve

DOTTED SWISS Lightweight fabric with embroiderylike designs of dots of various sizes. Achieved through a special weaving technique called clip spot weave. Also achieved through flocking, a surface effect of gluing the design to the fabric, generally less durable.

DOUBLE-BREASTED Front closure of garment with wider lap of fabric and two vertical rows of buttons, one row for buttoning and the other for decorative effect. There is usually an

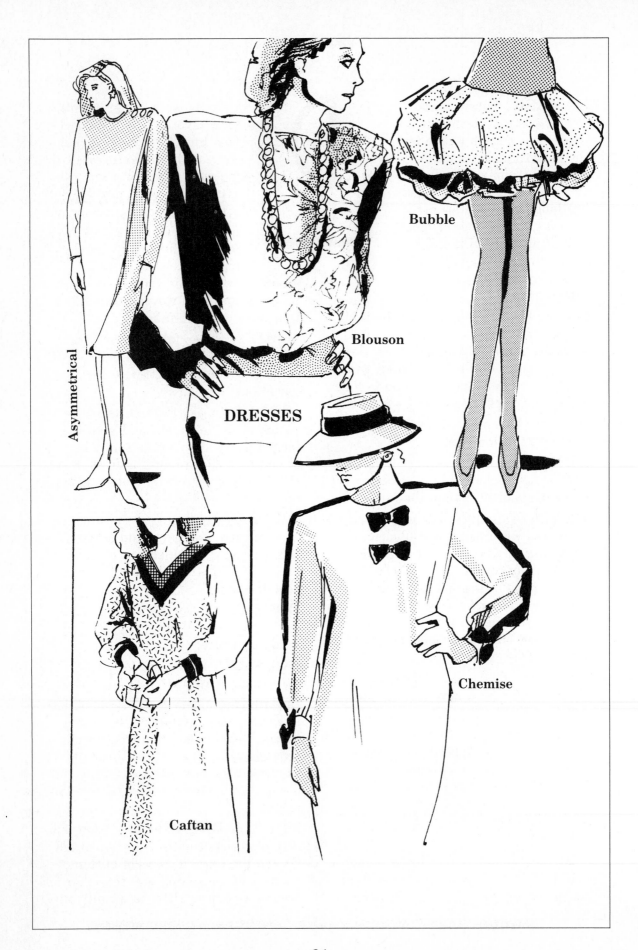

Asymmetrical

Bubble

Blouson

DRESSES

Caftan

Chemise

24

inside button used to hold the inner layer of fabric in place.

DOUBLE CLOTH Fabric woven with five yarns to produce a heavy, reversible fabric. May be of two colors. Used for coats, jackets, or capes.

DOUBLE-FACE SATIN A satin weave variation which gives both sides of the fabric a lustrous look.

DOUBLE KNIT A heavier, more durable knit, with less stretchability. Knitted with double needles. Popular in 1950's and 1960's. Still in use today, especially as a "pull on pant" for a segment of the female population.

DOUPIONI SILK Fabric from yarn of double cocoons. Has textured, slub effect. *see* Silk.

DOWN Soft feathers from ducks and other water fowl. Used for insulation in outerwear apparel.

DRAPE The way in which fabric hangs or falls into loose folds.

DRAPING Technique used by designers to create garments by draping fabric on dress form. A pattern is then cut from the draped segments and made into the designer's sample garment.

DRESS 1. To put clothes on, to set hair. 2. Clothing, one or two pieces, for women and girls, made of lighterweight fabrics, from simple to ornate designs. Synonymous for frock or gown.

The first version of the dress in ancient Egypt, was a rectangle, worn wound around the body. Dresses, referred to as "gowns" in Ancient Egypt became sheer, elaborately pleated rectangles. Cretan women's dress was primarily a bell or tiered skirt, accompanied with a snug fitting, breastrevealing blouse. The tunic was the basic garment of all Roman and Greek peoples, worn by both sexes. The female tunic was ankle length. This fashion continued for centuries.

Women of the Dark Ages wore a *stola*, a full gown with long, full sleeves, girdled about the waist, and of silk, wool, or linen fabric. A slim long dress was worn under this as an undergarment. The Medieval female garment was a floor length, slender, fitted dress with deep skirt slits and full sleeves. A decorative tassled belt completed the look. The twelfth century coat dress was termed a *Cotehardie*, with a fitted bodice and long gored skirt. It became excessive in width and was famous for the inverted "S" profile, giving the women a sway back, pregnant look.

Women of the Renaissance wore long, flowing decorative gowns, many elaborately ruffled, embellished and jeweled, and many with long trains. In France, Mme. de Pompadour and Mme. Du Barry were influential in promoting the most elegant styles of dresses of rich fabrics. The Watteau gown, of the Baroque Era was made with a fitted front bodice and huge, tentlike back, with an underdress. Following the French Revolution, the dress was a simple chemise of Empire styling and seamed under the breast.

A fashion dress of 1800 was formal looking and called Daytime Gown. Another, less formal was the Carriage dress. The dress of 1890 to 1910 was long, figure concealing, and of wool. Earliest sport use was the Bathing Dress of the early 1900's. The housedress of 1930's to 1960's was worn by women at home during the day to do housework. Current fashions include:

A-Line Dress with no waistline. Skirt flares from upper body to hem.

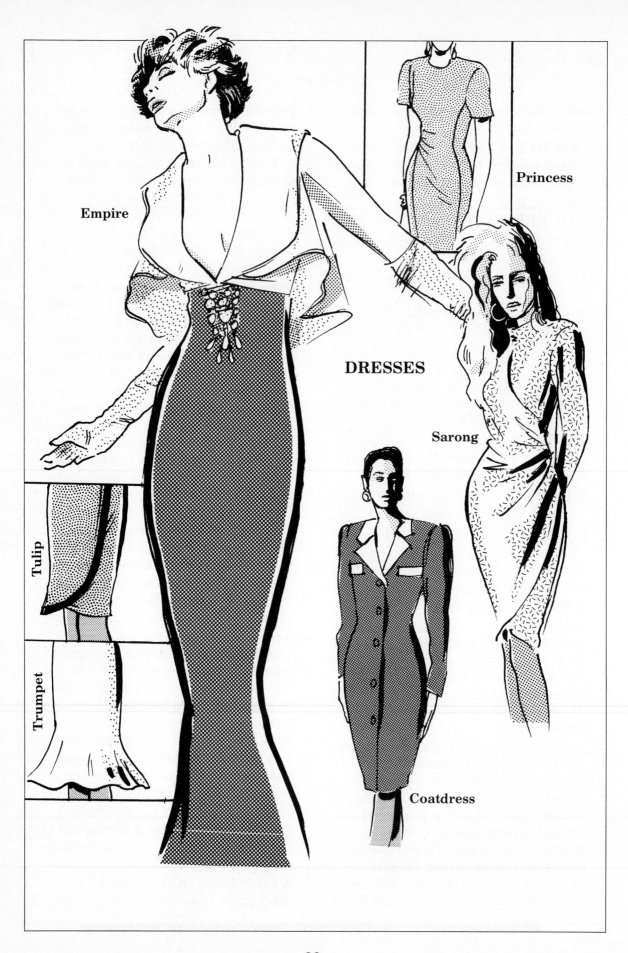

Empire

Princess

DRESSES

Sarong

Tulip

Trumpet

Coatdress

Asymmetric Dress with off-center closure or design elements.

Blouson One piece dress with bloused top sewn to waistline or to dropped waist seam of skirt.

Bubble Dress characterized by bubble or pouf skirt, the fullness of skirt attached to less full lining, with exterior appearance of a large bubble.

Caftan Full length dress of ethnic origin, with bell sleeve and embroidered neck and center opening area.

Chemise (sha mēz') One-piece, straight line dress with no waistline. Also called *sack dress*. Has had many variations.

Cheongsam (che ôŋ' säm') Long, straight chemise style dress with high thigh side slits and mandarin collar. Of Chinese origin.

Coat Classic, single- or double-breasted, notch collar dress with simple coatlike appearance. Sometimes belted.

Empire (äm pir') Dress with high waist seam just under the bust with a straight, gathered, or flared skirt. First introduced by Empress Josephine of France and revived several times since. *see also* Empire.

Formal More elegant dress for evening party or other special occasion.

Jumper One-piece dress without sleeves and with lower neckline, to be worn with blouse or sweater for sleeve and neckline contrast.

Little Black Classic, simply designed black dress, for all special occasions. Usually worn with jewelry to enhance the fashion look.

Muumuu Dress from Hawaii. Loose, full, bright floral design, in general style of smock dress.

Peasant Classic-styled dress with gathered round neckline, full bodice, and full gathered skirt. Sometimes with hem ruffles and full puffed sleeve.

Pinafore Bib top dress with shoulder ruffle and full gathered skirt. Originally designed to be an apron. Worn with a blouse.

Princess Classic-styled dress with vertical panels that fit to the body and flare in the skirt. Originated in France when Charles Worth designed this for Empress Eugenie. Also used as a classic coat style.

Sailor Dress with nautical look. Usually has a middy collar and braid.

Sari Fine fabric chemise with additional fabric that wraps at the waist and the loose end is placed over shoulder as a drape. When properly worn, it must be meticulously wrapped using exact directions. Of Hindu origin.

Sarong Strapless top dress with wraparound skirt and side drape. Of Indonesian origin.

Sheath Simple straight dress, somewhat fitted at waist using vertical darts.

Shirtwaist Tailored, elongated shirt becomes a dress with center front button closure. A classic style. May be belted, single- or double-breasted.

Smock Dress with top yoke. The gathered fabric of the skirt is sewn to the yoke. Often used as a maternity dress. From *painter's smock*.

Sundress Variety of styles: sleeveless, halter top, strapless, or with narrow shoulder straps. Worn in warm weather for comfort.

Surplice Dress with a wrapped, asymmetrical top, attached at waist seam to skirt of dress.

Sweater Elongated sweater worn as a one-piece dress or as a two-piece dress with lesser elongated sweater top and pencil narrow sweater knit skirt.

Tent Dress of the 1960's with triangular shape that flares from narrow shoulders.

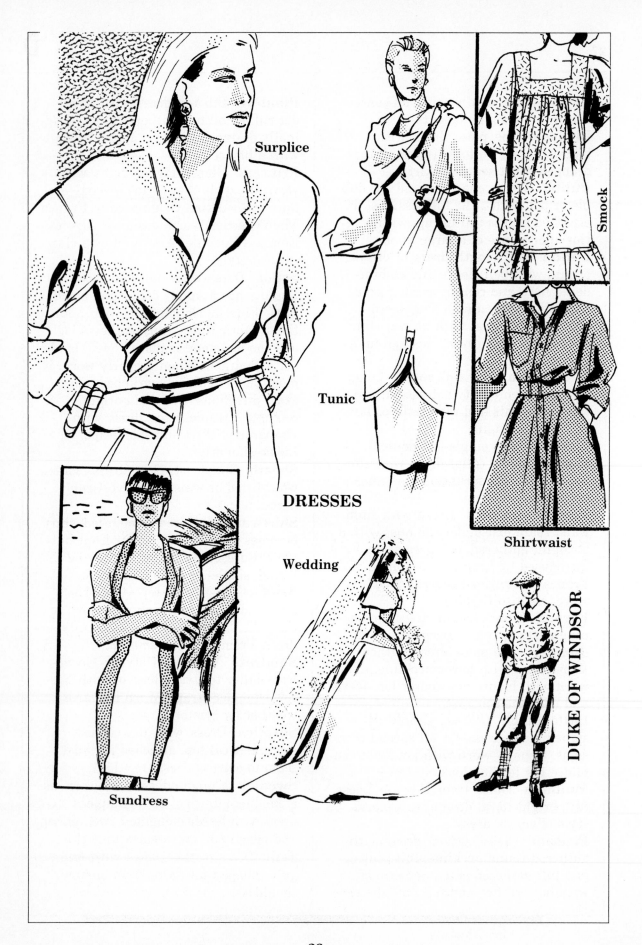

Surplice

Tunic

Smock

Shirtwaist

DRESSES

Wedding

Sundress

DUKE OF WINDSOR

Trapeze Silhouette with very full flared skirt similar to a tent dress. Introduced in 1950.

Trumpet Dress with wide circular flounce in skirt to resemble the top of trumpet.

Tulip Slim dress with wrapped skirt, resembling a tulip before the flower fully opens.

Tunic Long, plain sleeve, or sleeveless top worn over a skirt to give a dress effect. Originally a knee length garment worn by men and women. Of early Greek and Roman origin.

Wedding Dress worn by a bride for her wedding. More elegant, bouffant and with train for first wedding. Usually white or pastel. Is more sophisticated and without train for second wedding.

Wrap Robelike (kimono style) dress that has full front opening, wraps around body and is secured with belt or sash.

DRESS FORM Forms are in the shape of the human body and are usually padded with soft exterior so that dressmakers/designers can drape and pin fabric when designing garments. Dress forms come in standard ready to wear (rtw) fashion industry sizes. Custom dress forms can be acquired by dressmakers and adjusted to an individual client's body size, for one-of-a-kind garments.

DRESSMAKER One who makes one-of-a-kind women's clothing.

DRILL Strong, durable twill weave fabric, often made of cotton or cotton blends. Major uses include work clothes and sportswear, as well as household use.

D-RING Two D-shaped metal rings are used as a buckle fastening for a belt by interlacing the belt through one ring and overlapping into the second ring. Used with belts for sportswear apparel, pants, trenchcoats, and others.

DROPPED SHOULDER *see* Shoulder

DROPPED WAISTLINE Waistline seam that attaches bodice to skirt at a below normal waist area. Sometimes dropped to hip level and may be to thigh level, as seen in silhouettes from the 1920's.

DUCHESSE SATIN Smooth fabric of satin weave, with a plain back, lustrous satin face, and crisp texture.

DUCK Light to heavyweight, cotton fabric of plain weave. Lightweight duck has been popular for men's slacks and took on the name *ducks*. Also used as shoe uppers in a summer shoe called an *espadrille*.

DUKE OF WINDSOR Named after Edward VIII, King of England, who reigned for a brief period. A fashion leader of the 1920's, he was known for wearing brown suede shoes. He made popular the wearing of *plus fours* and *Fair Isle sweaters* for golf. Also known for popularizing the Panama hat and the tie with a broad knot named the Windsor knot. His favorie suit style, with padded wide shoulders and narrow fit over the hips, was widely copied.

DUNGAREE *see* Pants

DUSTER An unconstructed coat. With the beginning of the automobile age, women began wearing a white or buff colored coat to protect their clothes from road dust, thus the name *duster*. The name has continued to be a style of coat that is lightweight, flared, and tent style. *see* Coat.

DYEING To add color to fabrics and other materials used for apparel and accessories. Early origins were from natural sources such as berries, barks, grasses, etc. Present day dyes are of a synthetic source. Selection of dyestuffs for coloring fashion materials requires highly trained individuals who are knowledgeable about how each fiber/material will take the color, the crucial area of colorfastness, and how combinations of fibers will take the dye. Choosing fashion colors for various seasons is done by fashion industry leaders, with careful regard for saleability to the customers.

Yarn Dyeing The coloring of yarns before the fabric is constructed, done to achieve patterns such as plaids, checks, or stripes. For additional ways that fabrics and fashion materials acquire color and pattern. *see also* Printing.

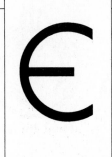

EARMUFFS 1. Two round circles of fabric, usually fleece or wool, approximately two inches in diameter, worn to keep ears warm in winter. Usually attached and held in place with band that goes over top of head. 2. Some winter caps have convertible ear covers (muffs) that can be extended down over ears or tucked inside cap when not needed for warmth.

EARRINGS Jewelry worn on the ear, made of precious metals and gems, semiprecious metals and gems, base metals, plastics, wood, stones, and other materials. Earrings were first worn by ancient Egyptians, as gold or silver dangles, hoop style with pottery stone insets, and pendant style. Earrings are noted in history as an accessory for men, either worn on one or both ears, and by women, typically as a set of two. Two main ways of attaching earrings to the ear: 1. clip: is affixed to back of earring, encircles earlobe and spring is used to maintain in place. 2. pierced: ears have had a small hole/s made through earlobe. A stud or post is inserted and a disk is attached on backside of lobe to hold in place. An alternative is a long curved wire, when inserted into hole, holds earring in place. Typical styles with many variations and prices include:

Ball A small, usually round earring of diamond, pearl, gold, or other material, that fits on earlobe. A double ball has a chain extension with a second ball that dangles at the end of the chain.

Button Usually larger and flatter than a ball, and fits on the end of the earlobe.

Cluster Multistones fastened to backing, worn on earlobes.

Doorknocker Longer, wider hoops, or other design, fitted onto an earpost and dangles free. Resembles a "house doorknocker," thus the name.

Drop An earring with chain attached and a second decorative ornament is attached and hangs free.

Hoop A circle, usually of a metal or plastic, that fits onto ear, or a larger, narrow circle that may dangle and is attached from a small button on earlobe.

Pendant A multidrop earring, usually of many stones or gems, used for elegant effect.

Post/Stud Part of earring, of gold or surgical steel, that goes through earlobe, for attachment on back side.

Shoulder Duster Very long, pendant style earrings.

EDGING Narrow, decorative, contrasting or multicolored trim, used on edge of areas of garment for decorative effect. Typical use on collar, yokes, cuffs, and neck edges.

EDWARDIAN A style of menswear clothing named for King Edward VII of England in the early 1900's. Dark colored suits with single-breasted coats, narrow lapels, and high buttoned on chest. Narrow trousers. Style revived in mid 1960's and again in the late 1980's by couture menswear designers.

EELSKIN *see* Leathers

EGYPTIAN SANDALS *see* Shoes

EGYPTIAN-STYLE Designs adapted from early Egypt, such as the tunic, sandals, collar necklaces, accordian pleating, massive jewelry, such as jeweled pendants and belts, wide gold bracelets, kilts (from early loincloth), cosmetics, and wigs.

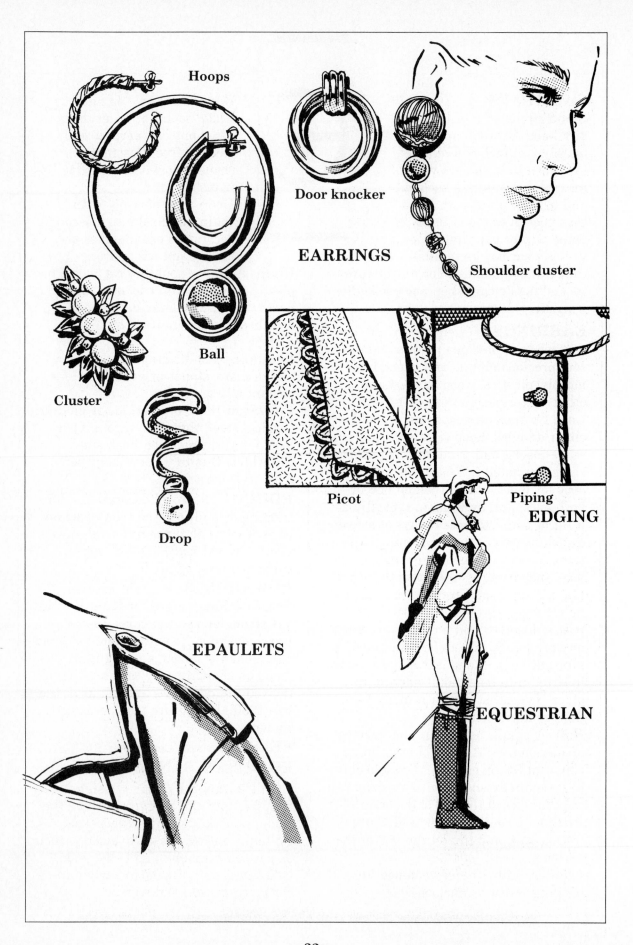

Hoops

Door knocker

EARRINGS

Shoulder duster

Cluster

Ball

Drop

Picot

Piping **EDGING**

EPAULETS

EQUESTRIAN

EISENHOWER A blouson jacket made famous when worn by General Dwight D. Eisenhower in World War II. *see* Jacket, Battle.

ELASTIC Stretchable fiber, originally a liquid from a rubber tree which was solidified. A manmade elastic fiber, named Spandex, was developed and introduced by DuPont in 1959 as Lycra. Both are used as core yarns, coverering the elastic with cotton or nylon. Rubber is in limited use and Spandex is widely used. Typically used for swimwear, underwear, skiwear, bodywear, sock tops, control top pantyhose, and some dress fabrics.

ELASTICITY Use of rubber or spandex to produce a product that expands and returns to shape and/or holds body in desired shape.

ELIZABETHAN Style of clothing and accessories from Queen Elizabeth I of England during the Renaissance in mid to late 1500's. Women's styles from this period included the lace ruff/collar (high lace cartwheel), large, round-hooped skirts, whalebone corsets, and jeweled hair and clothing. Men's styles included full leg hosiery and doublet, from which the current vest is fashioned.

EMBELLISHMENT Using ornamentation such as beading, sequins, appliqué, or embroidery to make part or all of garment more beautiful.

EMBOSSED Process of pressing a design, by use of heat and engraved rollers, onto a rather rigid material such as leather, metal, or fabric.

EMBROIDERY Needlework done by hand or machine to embellish or decorate fabric. First used in ancient Egypt by using fine gold wire to hand stitch designs on to royal apparel. Machine embroidery is done on a Swiss machine called a Schiffli. Hand embroidery is applied to fabric by use of a needle and contrasting, matching, or colored threads using stitches such as the cross stitch, chain stitch, satin, buttonhole, or hemstitch. These same stitches can be produced by machines.

EMERALD *see* Gems

EMPIRE (äm pir′) A style of women's apparel. Typically a dress, that fits the figure over the bust with a skirt which hangs from the seam below the bust resulting in a no-waist effect. Also called a *high-waisted chemise* from the French Empire period under the reign of Napoleon I in the 1800's. The Empire style includes a small woman's bonnet and Empire coat, a full-skirted, high waistline coat. *see* Dress, Empire.

ENGLISH DRAPE A man's suit jacket style of 1930's and 1940's with top fullness, nonfitted waist and tapering to hips.

ENSEMBLE (än säm′ b'l) A total look, including coordinating apparel and accessories. Of French origin.

ENVELOPE *see* Handbag

EPAULET/EPAULETTE (ep′ ə let′) An ornamental shoulder tab worn on military uniforms. Adapted to current fashion for a military look. A flat tab over shoulder, usually buttoned in place. Typically on raincoats/trenchcoats and other apparel. Of French origin.

EQUESTRIENNE (i kwes′ trē en′) Female horsewoman. Current equestrienne fashion ensemble includes visor cap, jacket, shirt, gloves, jodphurs, and boots. Of French origin.

ERMINE Elegant white hair fiber from animal of weasel family.

EROGENOUS (i räj′ə nəs) Theory of dress which states that sexual emphasis focuses on one part of the body and that clothes reflect this by exposing this area. Examples would be a low neckline exposing the breasts or a short skirt that exposes the legs.

ESPADRILLE *see* Shoes

ETHNIC Pertaining to fashions from different countries/races.

ETON (ēt′ ′n) A schoolboy look adapted from a prescribed outfit worn by students at Eton College in England in the 1800's. Includes close fitting, small visor cap, waist length jacket, vest, and trousers.

EUGENIE (yoo jē′ nē) Empress of France, wife of Napoleon III. Considered a foremost fashion leader. Established Charles Worth as her personal and court designer/couturier. The most important styling innovation of this time was Worth's Princess style gown, a dress with vertical panels, form fitting, with skirt flare, designed by Worth for Empress Eugenie.

EVENING Clothes worn for "after 5." More formal/dress occasions.

EXERCISE APPAREL *see* Bodywear

EYELET A fabric with holes punched out and embroidery, typically using buttonhole stitch, is worked around holes to produce the design. Can be done by hand or Schiffli machine. Also called Madeira—area where this was first begun.

FABRIC Cloth made from the yarn of a fiber. Yarns are transposed into fabric by several methods: weaving and knitting are the most commonly used methods, having many variations. Also, a non-woven method such as felt, and ornamental methods such as lace, braid and others are used.

FACE The outside or right side of the fabric.

FACET In jewelry, when cuts are made to the gemstone to reflect light and enhance beauty.

FACING An outer fabric piece sewn to a cut or unfinished edge of apparel and turned inside to "finish" the edge. Used at the neckline and sleeve areas, as well as closures.

FAD A fashion that is short-lived and very popular.

FADE Term used to describe the slow loss of color due to washing, exposure to sunlight, or other causes.

FAGOTING A method of decorating apparel by joining two pieces of fabric together with spaced thread bars. Can be done by hand or machine.

FAILLE (fil) Fabric of good body, ribbed, usually lustrous, and generally used for eveningwear.

FAIR ISLE *see* Sweaters

FALL A hairpiece, either of natural or imitation hair, added at the crown, to "fall" down over the back of the head.

FAN A decorative, pleated accessory item of paper or fabric. A hand held accessory, which, when in movement, creates a breeze of air for the holder.

FANNY PACK Colorful accessory that is worn around waist with a pouch to carry essentials. Worn by skiers, hikers, and by shoppers, not wishing to carry a handbag.

FANNY WRAP Use of cloth, brought around fanny to add design to apparel.

FASHION A style that is accepted and in use by a majority or group of people. To be "in fashion" is to wear the accepted style by a given group. "High fashion" denotes the wearing of designer apparel and a fashion forward appearance.

FASHION CYCLE The circle of a fashion item from Introduction, Rise, Culmination, Decline to Obsolescence. May then be reintroduced and the cycle repeats, which is typical of classic fashion apparel or accessories.

FASHION DOLLS Small dolls, dressed in the highest fashions of continental Europe, sent to England and other countries to communicate the newest fashion. First began in 1300 when an English queen sent a request to Europe for samples of a continental court dress. In the early days of America, fashion dolls were delivered by ship to major Eastern ports, dressed in the latest styles, complete with accessories and hair styles. Dolls were used to communicate fashion until the development of fashion magazines.

FASHION FORECAST Prediction by fashion forecasters of the direction in which fashion is going. The identification of trends and prediction of consumer acceptance of styles and colors.

FASHION GROUP, INTERNATIONAL, INC. World wide professional organization of women working in the Fashion Industry. First organized in 1931 in New York City. Regional groups were formed in the 1950's and recently the organization expanded worldwide. Membership now includes men.

FASHION IMAGE The mental representation or sensory picture an individual perceives of a store, object, garment, or person.

FASHION INDUSTRY All elements combined to design, produce, and sell fashion apparel and accessories.

FASHION MAGAZINES *see* Magazines

FASHION MERCHANDISING The planning, buying, and selling of fashion apparel and accessories to consumers.

FASHION PROMOTION The planning and production of special events which inform the consumer of fashion merchandise. Most popular event is a fashion show which uses models to wear the merchandise to show the customers. The shows are often reproduced and shown on video tapes or TV. Promotion also uses mannequins to promote merchandise, as well as seminars and other special events.

FASHION SHOW Used to promote a new season of fashions. Models display fashions to prospective customers. Three types of fashion shows: formal, in which models walk to music in a formal setting; production, using theaterlike vignettes or playful skits along with the display of fashions on models; and, informal, having a limited number of models to show fashions in an informal way to customers in a department of a store.

FASTENER A button, hook, snap, velcro, or other item used to close/secure an area of apparel or accessory. *see* Closure.

FAUX (fō) False, fake. Of French origin.

FEATHER Used to decorate garments, used for fans, or hair accessories. A Feather Boa is a long scarf worn over the shoulders, made entirely of feathers. The Marabou (species of stork) with fine feathers, the Osprey, with long feathers, the Ostrich with plumed feathers and long Peacock feathers are most commonly used. *see* Boa.

FEDORA *see* Hats

FELT Fabric created by use of matted fibers compressed into fabric by use of heat, moisture, and pressure. Felt is not considered firm or strong enough for apparel but is widely used in hats because it can be shaped and molded into various shapes and designs. Wool fiber was first used for felt, now other fibers are also used. The felt process is also used to make nonwoven interfacings and disposable hospital surgical apparel.

FIBER The base product used in making yarns. Two types of fibers: natural, from plant, animal, or mineral source; and manmade, manufactured from chemical source.

FIBERFILL Short fibers, usually of polyester, used as filler or insulation in outerwear, padded bras, and as the filler for quilted fabrics.

FILAGREE A fine thread of metal, usually gold or silver, applied to jewelry for ornamental, openwork designs.

FILAMENT Long fibers. All manmade fibers are extruded as filament fibers. Silk is the only natural filament fiber. All filaments can be cut into staple fiber. *see* Staple. Yarns can be monofilament (one) and multifilament (many). Monofilament is used for sheer hosiery. Filaments can be twisted, textured, made soft, and bulky, and heat set to produce a crimping.

FINDINGS Fashion industry term for small items used in the making of apparel, such as buttons, zippers, ribbon, and tape.

FINE JEWELRY Designation of the finest gemstones and metals. *see* Gemstones; Metals.

FINISHES The application or special process to give fabric a property to improve its appearance, wearability, or performance. Examples are permanent press, water repellancy, and many others.

FLANGE A wide fold of fabric, used over the shoulder/sleeve area for decorative effect.

FLANNEL A plain weave, soft fabric, achieved by slightly raising the fiber ends in the finishing process called *napping*. Fabric may be of wool, cotton, or other fiber. Considerable use in nightwear, childrenswear, and men's shirts.

FLAPPER Referring to the female look of the 1920's. The carefree, slim, shapeless, boyish silhouette with long waist, short skirt chemise and bobbed (short) hair. Female emancipation progressed swiftly after World War I when women had taken the place of men in industry. The new equality of the sexes changed society, allowing women greater independence, new dress and lifestyles. The short or long, tubelike, flat-chested dress was popular, use of make up, short bobbed hair, a passion for dancing, and disdain for conventional dress and behavior characterized the Flapper.

FLARE Adding fullness to a straight silhouette garment such as a skirt or pant so the lower area is wider than the top.

FLAX The plant source of the fiber, linen. The 2 to 4 feet stalk, after processing, produces linen fiber and the seed of the plant is used for linseed oil. *see* Linen.

FLEECE 1. A soft fabric produced by a pile weave or pile knit. The loops are cut to achieve the fleece effect. 2. The hair sheared from a sheep to be used for making wool.

FLOCKING/FLOCKED A finishing process that applies a design to fabric by pressing and glueing small yarns or dots for special design effect.

FLORAL A fabric with flower designs.

FLOUNCE A circularlike piece of fabric applied, usually, near the hem of a skirt, for design effect. *see* Dresses.

FORMAL Clothing worn for a special occasion, or After 5 events.

FOULARD (foo lärd′) Light weight twill weave silk with small design. Usual use, neckties. Of French origin.

FOUNDATIONS Undergarments for women, with additional support for body firmness. Garments such as support panties, pantyhose, girdles, and bustiers (Merry Widows). From the corset of earlier years.

FOX Animal related to a dog, with long fur. Raised on farms. Pelts are made into fur apparel and trims.

FRAGRANCES Pleasant, aromatic odor, or scent. Used in almost all cosmetic items from soap, lotions, and bath oils and in all forms of perfumes, toilet water, and colognes. Early users of fragrances rubbed flower petals on their bodies. Currently there are two methods of producing a fragrance: 1.

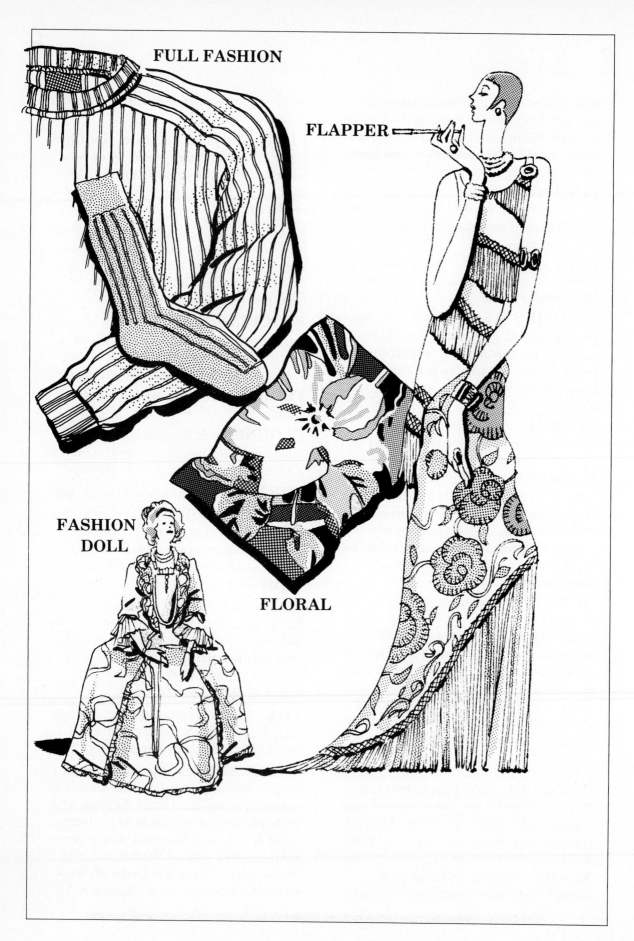

FULL FASHION

FLAPPER

FASHION
DOLL

FLORAL

essential oils are extracted from flowers, leaves, fruits, woods, and other sources. Fixatives are added to extend fragrance life. 2. synthetic fragrances are made from chemicals. Both methods are expensive and their formulas are secrets.

Perfume Contains the greatest amount of essential oils, slightly diluted with alcohol.

Eau de toilette (ōdə twə let) Contains a lesser amount of the essential oils, more alcohol, and distilled water for dilution.

Cologne Has the smallest amount of essential oils and is diluted the most. These are all priced accordingly, with colognes the least expensive. Many designers and well-known personalities have one or more fragrance with special names and elegantly designed containers.

FRENCH BRAID *see* Hairstyles

FRENCH TWIST *see* Hairstyles

FRINGE Decorative trim of hanging threads or narrow strips of fabric, leather, or beads. Can be attached separately to a garment.

FROCK Synonymous with dress. Term has been used since Medieval times with various meanings, to denote a variety of clothing: a painter's smock, a garment worn by sailors, or members of clergy. A frock coat, worn by men in the eighteenth century, was a fitted, buttoned, and full-skirted garment.

FROG Decorative fastener formed into a flowerlike design using braid or cording of fabric. Containing a loop to fit over a buttonlike knot of fabric. Of Chinese origin.

FULL-FASHIONED Knitted into the shape of the area of the body it covers. Examples: full-fashioned hose are knitted to the shape of the leg, full-fashioned sweaters, knitted to the form of the body.

FUR The hide of animal with hair intact, called the pelt. Processed by manufacturer for longevity and suitable for consumer use. Fur designers create apparel and accessories; and fur manufacturers produce the items for consumer purchase. Merchandising furs is done through specialty stores, leased departments in retail stores, or consignment selling. Furs have been a sign of nobility, wealth, and status since the beginnings of ancient civilizations.

Two laws of the twentieth century have protected the consumer and the animals. The Federal Fur Products Labeling Act of 1952 states that the consumer must be informed about the name of the animal, the country of origin, other processes used (shearing, dyed, etc.), and the use of paws and tails. Because of the possible extinction due to overzealous individuals, the 1973 Federal Endangered Species Act was passed. It forbids the import or transportation over state lines of a variety of animals or products made from certain animal fur. Over half of the furs used in the United States result from animals produced on fur farms.

Endangered species are protected in many countries by a limitation of the number of certain animals that can be killed. Greenpeace is the consumer advocate group protecting animals from industry/consumer use. Furs are used in full-length coats, jackets, as trim, as lining in coats and gloves, or as capes, called stoles. The most widely used fur in the United States is mink. Other popular furs are fox, ermine, lamb, lynx, and rabbit.

Faux Fur Use of manmade fibers, usually modacrylic/acrylic, to produce fur fabric that resembles animal fur, but without the "hand" of real fur. A popular price substitute or choice for those wishing the look of fur.

FUSED Manufacturers term for applying interfacing to outer fabric through the use of adhesive, heat, and pressure. Commonly used in collars, lapels, and front closures of garments to add stability. In manufacturing apparel the fused seam, though in limited use, is an alternative to the traditional manner of sewing seams.

G

GABARDINE Durable fabric of warp face twill weave. Made into a variety of weights and of different fibers: wool, rayon, cotton, and man-made fibers. Used in apparel such as pants and suits.

GAITER Dates back to early footwear. In the 1800's, was used to cover a man's ankle area and worn with slip-on type of shoe. In the late 1800's worn by women with low cut shoes, over the ankle area for warmth in cold weather or for sporting activities. Its current form is a wide strip of fabric used by skiers, especially cross-country type, to protect the ankle and lower leg from snow and cold.

GARMENT Any article of clothing.

GARMENT TRADE Synonymous for the Apparel Industry.

GARNET *see* Gemstones, semi-precious

GARTER 1. Elasticized band, often decorative, worn around the leg to support hose. Worn this way by men in the eighteenth century. 2. A suspenderlike strap with fastener on the end to attach and support hose. Worn by men in the 1930's with strap fastened around the calf to support socks. Garters attached to girdle or garter belt worn by women to support hosiery, before the advent of pantyhose. Now, a fashion item, colored, or black with lace, and decorative. 3. A decorative leg garter is often worn on one leg by brides today, to be removed by the groom after the wedding.

GATHERING/GATHERS An accumulation of cloth formed by drawing together threads in a row or rows of stitches.

GAUCHO (gou′ chō) A fashion term that describes a pant skirt. Of South American origin. *see* Culottes.

GAUNTLET A large cuffed glove of the seventeenth century.

GAUZE Plain and open weave, limp and low thread count fabric. Nondurable. Used for some women's apparel such as blouses and dresses.

GEM CUT Fashioning a rough gemstone into a specific shape for beauty and light reflection. The artisan cuts facets (flat faces) onto the stone, then grinds and polishes it. Gem cuts include the following:

Baguette A rectangular cut.

Brilliant Cut Fifty-eight facets is the finest cut with the best light reflection. Other cuts vary from 18 to 58 facets.

Emerald Cut Rectangular with rounded corners, to bring out the finest color in colored stones.

Marquise (mär kēz′) Oval cut with end points.

Pear-shape A round end and a pointed end, looking something like a pear.

GEMS, MANMADE Zirconia, the look of a diamond.

GEMSTONES Precious or semi-precious stones that, when cut and polished, are used as jewelry and adornment. Precious gemstones include diamonds, rubies, sapphires, emeralds, and some pearls. Precious gemstones are described as the following:

Diamond The king of gems. A form of pure carbon and the hardest substance known. Varies in color from blue, yellow, pink, to clear. The value depends on the color, clarity, cut, and carat weight. The finest diamonds are

41

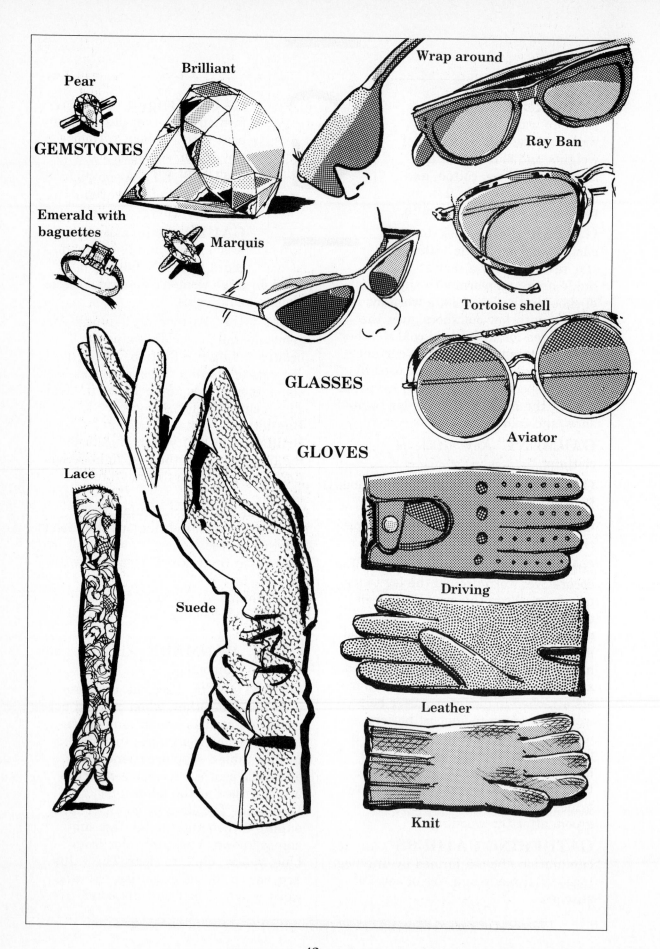

Pear

Brilliant

GEMSTONES

Emerald with baguettes

Marquis

Wrap around

Ray Ban

Tortoise shell

GLASSES

Aviator

GLOVES

Lace

Suede

Driving

Leather

Knit

42

brilliant cut. Diamonds are also used industrially.

Emerald A rich, green gemstone of the beryl family. The color of the emerald is from traces of chromium. Fine quality emeralds may be as costly as diamonds. Value is determined by color, flawlessness, and size.

Ruby and Sapphire Both are from the corundum species, an oxide of aluminum. Red is known as the ruby. Other corundum having colors other than red are known as sapphires (denotes blue). Colors vary from blue, white, yellow, and pink and vary by the presence of traces of iron. The finest quality of sapphire is a rich blue. A star sapphire, with starlike asterism, is caused by inclusions.

Semiprecious gemstones are described as the following:

Amber The fossilized resin of ancient trees. Hard, translucent yellow, orange, or brownish-yellow.

Amethyst Transparent quartz, with a color from pale violet to deep purple.

Aquamarine From the beryl family. Transparent blue to blue-green color.

Carnelian A variety of chalcedony. Clear, pale red to deep red.

Chrysoberyl Yellow-brown to blue-green. Varieties include Alexandrite; red to green color depending upon light source; and Cat's-eye, a chabochon variety. When cut, the band of light resembles a cat's eye.

Citrine Pale yellow variety of quartz, also in other colors.

Coral The calcified secretion of a marine animal. Commonly pink to orange color. Varieties of colors including black.

Garnet Silicate minerals with a vast color range. Typically pink to deep red. More opaque than the ruby. Colors vary from red to brown and blue.

Jade From two unrelated minerals: nephrite and jadeite. Jadeite is the rarer of the two and more highly prized, from Burma. Nephrite is more common. Jade occurs in many colors: white, green, yellow, red, and black. Used in necklaces, but is also an excellent material when carved into jewelry items.

Jet From hard coal, black, and polishes well. Popular mourning jewelry in the Victorian era.

Lapis Lazuli Opaque, azure blue to deep blue, from the mineral lazurite.

Moonstone Pearly, translucent mineral. From feldspar.

Onyx A chalcedony that occurs in bands of colors, especially used for cameos because of the veins of colors. Popular use of black for all types of jewelry.

Opal Softest of the more popular gems. Brilliant colors are due to impurities (inclusions). Opals are white to black. Fire opals have more inclusions and more color, opals are very brittle. There are no old or ancient opals due to the ease of cracking and breaking. Opals carry a common mystique of bringing good luck to those born in October and who wear opals as their birthstone.

Pearl (Cultured) Smooth and lustrous. Created by the secretion of the mollusk (oyster) over an irritant such as a grain of sand or other foreign matter. The value of pearls depends on shape, color, and size. The highest value is given to pearls that are large, white with pink, yellow-tinged, round and free of blemishes.

Quartz Brilliant and abundant hard crystal. *see* Amethyst; Citrine.

Topaz Crystal, usually in shades of yellow. When cut and polished, is very brilliant. Also found in blue, brown, or pink, but is more rare.

Turquoise Opaque stone, colored blue to green. Finest quality is of deep blue. More popular and abundant is green color. A porous stone. May be waxed or oiled to improve color.

Zircon Colorless, with brilliance and look of a diamond. Because of the lower hardness it chips easily. Also found in other colors: brilliant blue, red, and green.

GENERIC In the fashion industry, the classification of basic fibers, either natural or man-made, that exist in their natural state or similar chemical composition state. The list was established by the Federal Trade Commission and named the Textile Fiber Products Identification Act (TFPIA). The law, effective March 3, 1960, provided for generic fiber content labeling in all textile products. The manufacturer may add its specific trademark. Example: Dacron® polyester.

GEOMETRIC DESIGN Use of designs, such as squares, triangles, oblongs, and circles to form designs on fabric and apparel.

GEORGETTE A sheer silk, or silklike fabric, made with highly twisted or creped yarns. Used in apparel such as blouses, dresses, and eveningwear.

GIBSON GIRL The shirtwaist blouse/dress fashion of the early 1900's. Charles Dana Gibson, American fashion illustrator of the 1900's, created the elegant fashion illustrations of women of this era. Of particular popularity of this time were women illustrated in the shirtwaist, which became known as the Gibson Girl.

GINGHAM Medium weight fabric, usually cotton or cotton blend, with small woven squares, alternating in two colors.

GIRDLE 1. From early Greek, a belt or sash wound around and encircling the waist. 2. Earliest Greek figure control, the "strophian," were bands of cloth wound about the body, under the bust, and over the waist and hip. The figure controlling corset/girdle was developed during the Renaissance. It has been in and out of style since. 3. The full corset, that was so restrictive of the early 1900's, developed into a waist to thigh garment. In present use, the garment has reinforced areas to control the stomach and hips. It can be pulled on or made with a side opening zipper or lacing for easier entry. Boning is available in some girdles for more control. Front and back garters are attached for hosiery. Also available in a long leg, half-thigh version, and as a brief with cotton crotch and leg garters. A lesser reinforced girdle is a pant liner, an all-in-one girdle and brief of nylon and spandex. 4. Girdles are prescribed by doctors for certain back problems and are obtained from medical supply sources.

GLASSES/EYEGLASSES Use of a lens or lenses to aid vision. Tinted sun glasses are a fashion accessory. Several frame styles made popular by consumer acceptance and long use are half (granny) glasses, small oval wire or plastic frames; aviator, worn by military pilots, is a full size lens with a horizontal rim on the top. Other styles have full or partial wire frames, or styles with clear or tinted plastic frames. John Lennon, of Beatles fame, in the 1960's made popular the round wire rim, again in fashion in the late 1980's.

Bifocal An eyeglass with two lenses in one glass, made for two vision problems. The vision dividing line can be made invisible.

Goggles Protective glasses, fully covering the eyes. Used in industry, sports, and aviation.

Trendy Glasses that make their appearance every few years. Of unusual shapes, colors, frames, or other decor.

GLENPLAID *see* Plaids

GLOVES A fitted covering for the hand, having a separate section for each finger and thumb. A fashion accessory worn for decor, warmth, or a firmer grip while driving. Made from leather, plastics, fabrics, or a combination of materials. Linings may be added for warmth. The slip-on glove of leather is worn for a fashion look. Usually extends to just above the wrist. Driving gloves usually have knitted or a stretch fabric outer area and leather or vinyl grip sections. Many higher priced cars have accessory selling departments and sell the "name" glove to wear while driving that particular car—a status symbol.

Gloves are used for almost all sports and have become designed for a fashion look as well. Gloves of lace and other special fabrics are an accessory for weddings. The opera glove is a long, arm length glove worn with eveningwear.

GOATSKIN Tough, pebble-grained leather from a goat.

GODET (gō-dāy) Triangular inset(s) sewn into the lower edge of a skirt for design effect and added fullness. Of French origin.

GODEY'S LADY'S BOOK Famous American fashion periodical of the 1800's, published by Louis Antoine Godey.

GOLD *see* Metals, Precious

GOLD LEAF Extremely thin, pure gold.

GOLD-PLATED *see* Metals, Electroplate

GONDOLIER'S HAT *see* Hat

GORDIAN KNOT Intricately tied square knot, originated by King Gordius of Phrygia. Decorative use in fashion today.

GORE Design term for sections of a skirt, wider at the hem than at the waist area, thus creating a flared look. There may be four, six, or more gores in a skirt design.

GORE-TEX® Man-made fabric that is waterproof, breathable, and windproof. Pores nearest the body pass moisture out through the Gore-Tex membrane that is hydrophobic, but does not let outside moisture, such as snow and rain, or wind, through to the body. Extensive use in outerwear.

GOSSAMER Soft, sheer, delicate fabric.

GOWN 1. Woman's dress, more formal in style. 2. Long, flowing garment, as a robe or nightgown. 3. Outer robe worn by scholars or clergy on formal occasions.

GRADING The process of adding or decreasing areas of the sample size pattern to develop smaller and larger pattern sizes.

GRAIN 1. The lengthwise or warp yarns of fabric. To be off-grain is to have distortion in the appearance of a garment. 2. The distinguishing marks on leather acquired when hair or feathers are removed.

GRASS CLOTH Term for fabrics made of grasslike plants such as hemp or ramie.

GREEK FISHERMEN'S CAP *see* Caps

GRIPPER *see* Closures

GROMMET A reinforced ring or eyelet through which a fastener can be passed.

GROSGRAIN (grō grān′) An obvious rib weave fabric, using more yarns to obtain the rib, or a thicker yarn to obtain the rib. Usually manufactured as ribbon and used for surface decoration, ribbons for the hair, or as a fabric belt/sash. Also used in millinery as the inner hatband. Of French origin.

GROS POINT A type of lace.

GUARD HAIR The smaller length hairs that protect and warm the body of a longer haired animal.

GUSSET Small square or triangle insert of fabric, sewn in the underarm area to give greater arm movement in the garment. Also used as inserts in handbags and shoes.

H

HABERDASHERY A dealer of men's furnishings, such as hats, shirts, or socks.

HABIT A distinctive type of dress: 1. religious order apparel; 2. horseback riding apparel.

HACKING SCARF A long scarf popularized by the Prince of Wales. A fad of college students of the 1930's.

HAIR DO/STYLE The style in which a woman's or man's hair is arranged. *see* Coiffure.

HAIR FIBERS The hair of a number of different animals, woven or knitted into fabrics and apparel. Fibers from sheep are most commonly used, dating back to 2000 to 3000 B.C. Sheep are sheared for the fiber whose characteristics are elasticity, crimping, resilience, absorbency, fire resistance, water repellancy, and warmth. Specialty fibers include the soft hair from the cashmere goat of India, China and Tibet; the soft, light brown hair fibers from the Bactrian camel of Asia; the fine, silky mohair fiber from the angora goat; the fine strong hairs from the alpaca of South America; the fine lustrous black and brown hair fibers of the llama of the South American Andes Mountains; the white soft, silky fiber of the angora rabbit; the hair fiber of the grey rabbit; and some rare, costly hair fiber of the vicuna, an undomesticated animal from South America.

HAIRSTYLES From earliest days, men and women took care of their head and hair. In ancient Egypt, they shaved their heads and wore wigs of natural hair or wool—a practice of cleanliness. This practice subsided and other civilizations, such as the Greeks, had their hair styled in curls and ringlets. The Romans wore short, curled hair. Medieval women wore their hair hanging free or braided, often with veiling concealing their hair. Renaissance hairstyles for men changed to shoulder length bobs. High Renaissance women wore their hair pulled back and covered with a type of hood.

Seventeenth century hairstyles began simple and became very elaborate with higher and higher pompadours, using false hair, wire frames, and many other embellishments to achieve the look. Men often wore a powdered, curled, or pigtailed wig. From this most elaborate era, the styles changed many times. Hairstyles from the 1950's to the present include:
Afro Round, big, permed hairstyle to look like Afro-American hairstyle.
Asymmetrical Off-center hairstyle, dissimilar on either side.
Beatle cut Longer hairstyle for men, with sideburns, and copying the early look of the English rock music group called The Beatles.
Beehive A high bubble resembling a beehive, achieved by backcombing hair and twisting around into a domelike look of a beehive.
Bob Short hair style of the 1920's, made famous by Coco Chanel.
Bouffant Backcombing hair to achieve an exaggerated fullness.
Braids One, two, or more, achieved by braiding with 3 multistrands of hair together. Sometimes worn straight down or wound around the head.
Buzz To shave areas or all of the head to a very short length.
Chignon (shēn′ yän) Hair is rolled into a circle at the lower back of the head.

Cornrows Hair is braided into many, many, narrow plaits; from African style.

Crew cut Men/boys very short haircut, so that the top hair stands straight up. Has been adopted as a female style, also.

Dreadlocks Long hairstyle with many multibraids. Of Jamaican origin.

Falls Addition of artificial long hair, to "fall" over shorter hair.

Feather cut Hair is cut in layers for a curly look. Made famous by the movie star, Farrah Fawcett.

French braid Hair is braided, starting at the top of the head, and going down the back by adding more strands at each braid, to achieve a spinelike look.

French Twist Hair is combed to back of head and made into a rectangular roll.

Mohawk Adapted from an American Indian hairstyle. Sides and back of head are shaved of hair, leaving a two inch or more high strip of hair at the center of the head.

Pageboy Shoulder length hair with ends curled under.

Pigtails Two side braids hanging down, frequently a young girl's hairstyle.

Pompadour Hair is styled by being brushed up high and smooth from forehead toward back. Of French origin.

Ponytail Hair is pulled to center of back of head and held in place with decorated elastic or rubber band. Resembles a pony's tail.

Punk Usually a version of the Mohawk, may be multi-colored. Center strip may be tall and spiky looking.

Queue As worn by the Chinese. A long, single braid hanging down back of head. In current fashion, a long, narrow, usually curly strand of hair hanging down at nape of neck.

Sassoon A short, straight boylike hairstyle for women, designed by Vidal Sassoon in Great Britain in the 1960's. Became a popular hairstyle in the United States.

Shag A long, nonstyled, layered, uncut look of a shaggy dog. Popular for men in the 1960's.

Shingle Manlike hairstyle for women. Popular in the 1960's.

Topknot Longer hair is styled by combing hair to the top of the head and winding hair into a circlelike knot, secured with hair or bobby pins.

Wash and wear Longer permed hair is washed and air dried to achieve a very curly look. Often moussed for a wet look.

Wedge Back of hair is cut from neck upward into a V-like wedge/shape.

HALF A part of something approximately equal to the remaining part. Used in fashion as in half glasses, half slip, half lining, etc.

HALF SIZES Women's dress sizes for shorter women with fuller bodies. Typically run from 12½ to 26½.

HALL OF FAME A three time award winner of the Coty is placed in the Coty Hall of Fame. *see* Coty.

HALTER *see* Neckline

HAND The feel of the fabric to one's hand, such as smooth, rough, soft, or stiff.

HANDBAG Also called bag or purse. The modern handbag has become a container for a multitude of personal possessions for women. Handbags are used by men in other countries, but are not as common in the United States.

A handbag is a fashion accessory that reflects one's style and personality. Early handbags were noted in the Greek period as a circle or square,

HANDBAGS

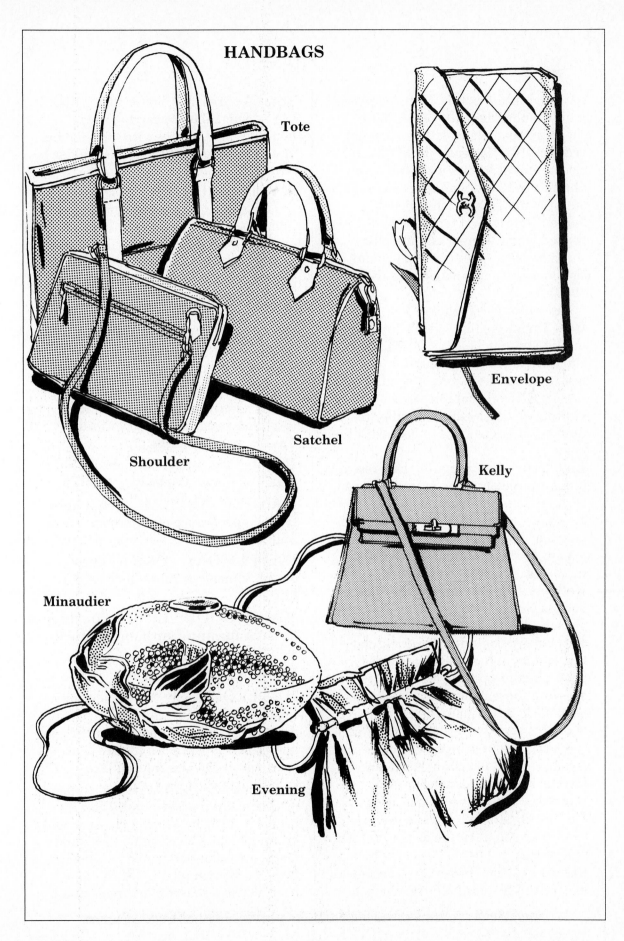

Tote

Envelope

Satchel

Shoulder

Kelly

Minaudier

Evening

49

gathered into a pouch. Many were ornately embroidered. By the 1700's, they had been elevated to an elegant accessory. By the early 1900's, snap-closing metal frames were developed, and in the 1920's, handbags were made out of many fabrications, including leather, fabric, and tapestry, and beaded, embroidered, and metallic small bags for evening. The popular shoulder strap bag dates from the 1950's.

Current styles include:

Box Rigid, boxlike with a top opening lid and handle.

Carpet Bag A bag, made from heavy carpetlike fabric. A smaller version of a travel container of the 1860's.

Clutch A bag with no handle, requiring the individual to hold with the hand.

Envelope A rectangular bag resembling a large envelope with a foldover closure, as in an envelope.

Evening Small, ornate, beaded, embellished bag used for special and/or evening occasions. Sometimes called minaudieres. (min od ee air)

Kelly A bag designed by Hermés for actress Grace Kelly.

Pouch Drawstring, circlelike bag.

Satchel A bag with a rectangular flat bottom and curved, rigid sides with a center opening and handles for carrying. Resembles a doctor's bag from early days. Many designers have used this style with their logos as patterns on the outside. May be of leather or fabric with a plastic coating and leather sides and handles.

Shoulder Any type of bag with varying length straps, to be carried over one's shoulder. Some have detachable straps.

Signature Any bag with a designer's logo or initials used all over the bag.

Tote A large bag, more utilitylike than fashionable, to carry a great many items. Usually with two handles, and may have a detachable shoulder strap.

HANDKERCHIEF A small square of fabric, usually cotton or linen, used to wipe one's nose or mouth. Often decorated with embroidery or lace and carried for special occasions. Men's handkerchiefs are larger and may be monogrammed with the individual's initials. *see also* Hem.

HANDKERCHIEF LINEN Sheer, soft linen used for blouses or dresses.

HAND KNIT The use of knitting needles and yarn by the individual to construct sweaters, baby clothing, dresses, or accessories.

HANG The way in which clothing hangs or fits on the body.

HANGER APPEAL Retail term for the appearance of a garment on a hanger in a store.

HAPPI COAT A hip or knee-length kimona or robe. Of Japanese origin.

HARD GOODS/LINES Industry term for furniture, appliances, televisions, etc. *see also* Soft goods/lines.

HAREM *see* Pants.

HARLEQUIN 1. A typical clown-type costume with eye mask, neck ruffle, and multicolored blocks on the top and tights. 2. Eyeglass frames that flare upward at the sides of face.

HARPER'S BAZAAR A women's fashion magazine (originally Bazar) begun in 1867 by Fletcher Harper and brothers, featuring fashion news and feature articles. Of primary interest were its fashion plates, which came from Berlin's counterpart magazine,

Der Bazar, that featured the latest in European fashion reported to the readers of *Harper's Bazaar*. The magazine was purchased by William Hearst in 1913 and continues today.

HAT A covering for the head, usually consisting of a crown to cover the head and a brim or edge extension. Headwear existed from the earliest days, and varied from fabric head coverings to head bands.

Historians believe that the hat was introduced into Europe by the Cretans, with many shapes, such as cones, turbans, tall, pointed crowns, and embellished, decorative trims. Men of early Greece wore a felt head covering with a brim which tied under the chin. The felt Pileus was a tall-crowned skull cap, common to all ancient people. Women of ancient Rome wore the Petasus, a straw sun hat. Medieval women's headwear included veils and wimples, which was a combined head, neck, and shoulder cover; chinstraps over cornets; and the fancy hennin, a very tall pointed cone. The Renaissance featured balzos for women, a large dome shape that completely covered the hair; and wigs and the Mary Stuart cap. Men of the Baroque era wore the high crowned beaver hat. Men and women wore hats, both indoors and out, as fashion accessories. They were highly decorated and trimmed. The elegance of the 1700's had men wearing the tricorn, with the brim pointed in three places. Women of this time had high, towering hairstyles and seldom wore hats.

After the French revolution, men's hats had become bicorn (2 creases) and women wore turbans or straw bonnets. Men's fashions of the 1800's continued to feature the top hat and women wore a variety of bonnets. Women of the early 1900's wore large brimmed decorated hats, often called Gainsborough, over high pompadoured hair. The women's hat of the 1920's was the famous cloche, a hair concealing hat, close fitting, over short hair. The turban was also worn, and men wore the fedora, boater, and Homburg. Since the 1940's, women's hats were small, sometimes cocked over one eye, small brimmed turbans, and the pillbox, made famous in the 1960's by Jacqueline Kennedy.

Since the 1960's hats have not been the fashion accessory they had been, either with men or women. Some fashionable women continue to wear hats. Styles are now worn by many for certain recreational activities, or to shade the sun, or protect from rain. Women's hats in London continue to be of great importance because of the use of hats by Queens and Princesses of the British family.

Alpine A colored fedora, adapted from authentic Swiss-German-Austrian Alps.

Beret (bə rā′) A soft circle of fabric shaped into a cap. Of French origin.

Boater/Skimmer A flat crown, wide flat brim hat, usually of straw. First worn by men in the 1920's.

Bowler/Derby A man's hat with high rounded crown and narrow, rolled up brim.

Breton A woman's hat with medium rolled-back brims, worn off the face.

Bush Men's hat with one side brim turned up. Originally worn by Australian soldiers in World War II.

Cartwheel/Halo Women's wide brimmed hat worn off the face.

Cloche Tight fitting, women's hat, some with narrow brims. Made famous in the 1920's.

Cowboy A large-brimmed leather hat with creased crown; used as a sun

HATS

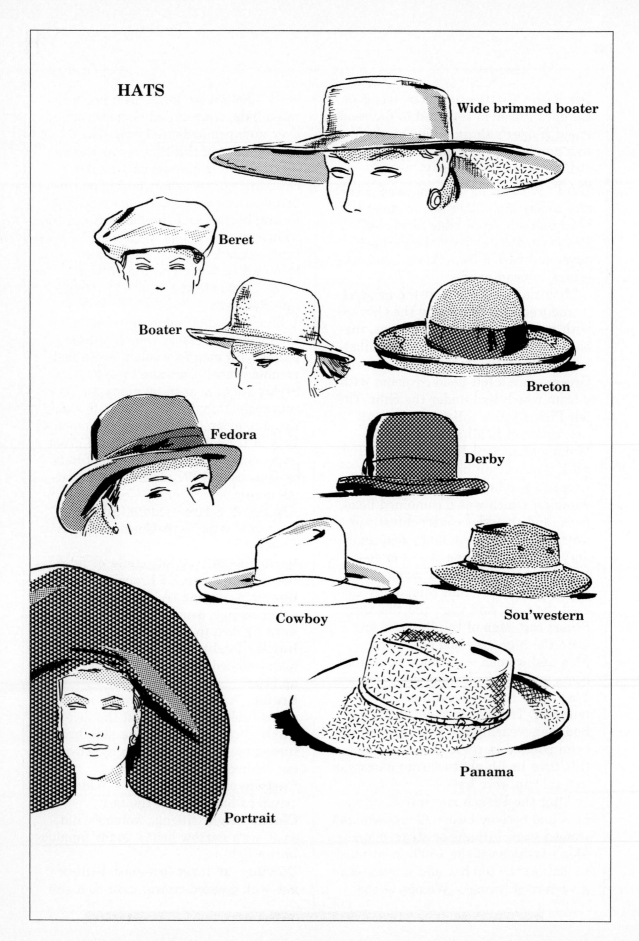

Wide brimmed boater

Beret

Boater

Breton

Fedora

Derby

Cowboy

Sou'western

Portrait

Panama

protecter. Sometimes called a ten-gallon hat.

Fedora Medium size man's hat with creased crown and slightly turned up brim. Brim may be tipped down in front, as the wearer chooses. Also worn by women.

Gaucho A boater-type hat, fastened under the chin by leather thongs or laces.

Gainsborough Monumental, large, decorated hats worn by women at the turn of the century over high pompadoured hair.

Hard Hat Hard metal or plastic hat used to protect the head when individual is in certain hazardous work areas.

Homburg Man's felt hat with soft, creased crown and shallow, rolled brim. First manufactured in Homburg, Germany.

Panama Natural-colored hat, handmade leaves from the jipijapa plant of Central and South America. Made famous in the 1920's by the Prince of Wales.

Picture/Portrait Women's hat with a large brim, to frame the face.

Pillbox Women's round, full crown, brimless hat. Made famous in the 1960's by Jacqueline Kennedy.

Planters Man's wide, rolled brim hat of straw, worn for protection from the sun.

Rain/Sou'wester First worn by fishermen. Hat with a large back brim, the front brim often turned up, to give protection from the rain.

Russian Fur A brimless fedora-type hat worn for warmth.

Sailor Small, narrow nautical hat with high upturned brim.

Sombrero Broad-brimmed Mexican or Spanish hat of felt or straw, to protect from sun.

Tam-o'-shanter A wide, flat beret with puff tassel on top.

Top Men's formal hat with high, stiff crown, and narrow brim.

Tote Men's protective rain hat of fabric with small turned down brim.

Turban Fabric wrapped or draped female hat, fully covering the head.

HATBAND Narrow ribbon or band of cloth, placed around a hat just above the brim, for decorative effect.

HAUTE COUTURE (ōt ko͞o tür') Means high fashion. The top designers' finest work. Of French origin. *see* High Fashion.

HEADBAND Band, usually ornamental, worn around head or over forehead.

HEAD WRAP Scarf worn around one's head.

HEATHER Greyish-purple color, from the color of a flowering shrub.

HEAT REFLECTIVE FINISH Method of providing additional insulation to fabric by spraying a coating of metal and resinous substance to back of fabric.

HEAT SET Some man-made fibers are treated with heat to set a permanent shape to prevent shrinkage. Sets in pleats, creases, or other permanent shaping.

HEAT SET YARN STRETCH In the manufacturing of man-made yarn, a crimping of the yarn by heat, enables yarn to stretch and return to its original shape.

HEAT TRANSFER PRINTING Dry printing process which uses a pre-patterned colored paper to transfer a design to most any fabric by a simple hot transfer operation of rolling paper and fabric together under pressure and high temperature.

HEEL The built up portion of a shoe or boot that supports the heel of

HEELS

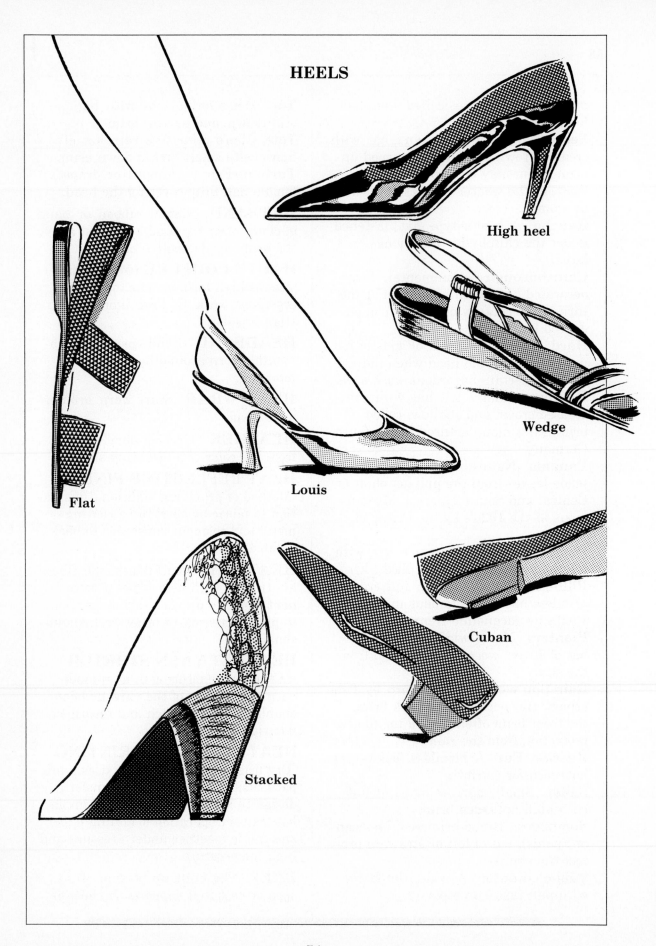

High heel

Wedge

Flat

Louis

Cuban

Stacked

the foot. First placed on shoes in the 1600's. Various types include: wide or chunky heel of the 1960's; stacked heel with the look of horizontal cuts of wood; Louis heel, a copy of the look of the Louis era, a heel which flares out near the bottom of the heel; current fashion heels of high, medium, and low heights; and the all-in-one wedge heel that is a heel that fills in the instep area, all in one piece.

HELMET Protective head covering of leather, metal, or plastic.

HEM To finish the raw or cut edge of fabric by rolling it to the back side and stitching into place. Various hems include: asymmetric, a hem that is longer in one area than another; handkerchief, a hem that falls into many triangular points, with the appearance of the use of handkerchief points; petal, a hem with lower edge hemmed in rounded sections; plain, the use of seam tape to finish off or cover raw edge of fabric and sewn to garment; rolled, a narrow hem, turned or rolled to back of fabric and sewn by hand or machine; shirt hem, narrow hem, turning raw edges to back side and machine stitched.

HEMP Very strong fiber obtained from the stem of a plant from the mulberry family. Major use is for twine or rope. Limited use in apparel.

HENLEY Men's collarless knit shirt with placket front.

HENNA Reddish-brown color from the leaves of an Asian/African tree. Used as a cosmetic dye and coloring for leather.

HERRINGBONE Decorative design that looks like a series of V's, achieved by the use of a right and left twill weave.

HIDES Animal skins over 25 pounds, used in leathermaking.

HIGH FASHION Styles that are accepted and worn by fashion leaders, usually among the first to accept the change to a new fashion. *see also* Haute Couture.

HIGH-RISE WAISTLINE Higher than the usual waistline.

HIP-HUGGER Lower than usual waistline, usually resting on hip bones. Popular in the 1960's in the design of pants and shorts.

HIPPIE Members of nonconformist groups, usually withdrawn from mainstream society and characterized by unconventional clothing, personal appearance, and living habits. From the mid 1960's.

H-LINE A straight, or H silhouette of the mid 1950's.

HOMBURG *see* Hats

HOMESPUN Heavier, coarser, plain weave fabric, originally from the terminology, "being made at home." Currently manufacturer's name for that "look" of fabric.

HONEYCOMB Use of a Dobby weave to produce a piqué fabric with a small honeycomb or waffle effect.

HOOD Loose covering for the head, attached to a jacket, coat, or robe.

HOOK AND EYE *see* Closures

HOOP Circular band. Hoop earrings—bands of metal or plastic. Hoop skirts—bands of plastic attached to a full skirt for a belled-out look.

HORIZONTAL FLOW THEORY Theory that fashions are adapted and move horizontally between groups of people on similar socioeconomic levels.

HORIZONTAL INTEGRATION Firms that merge or take over other firms with the same function.

HORSEHAIR Hair fiber from the horse. In past fashion, used for braids in millinery or dressmaking. Little use in apparel today.

HOSE/HOSIERY Stockings or socks used as covering for foot and legs. Men first wore tube hose in the 1100's. These were folded rectangles, cut and sewn to fit the foot and leg. This was followed by leg-shaped fabric cut and sewn together. Used by men in this form for many centuries. Became decorative, often multicolored.

Knitting techniques became perfected in the 1500's by the invention of the knitting machine by William Lee. By the 1600's hose had become more decorative, made of linen, or silk with lace cuffs. Both men and women were now wearing hosiery, however, women's were hidden by their long skirts. By the 1920's, with the development of the fiber rayon, hosiery for women was being made in both rayon as well as silk.

The development of nylon and its manufactured use for hosiery, introduced in 1939, revolutionized hosiery for women. Most all hosiery worn by women today is of nylon fiber. There are nylon/spandex blends which give more tummy and/or leg support and there are some with the addition of cotton in the crotch. There are small numbers of hosiery made from 100 percent cotton.

Current styles of female hosiery include: ped, a foot cover; anklets, only ankle high; knee high; thigh high, not needing garters and thigh highs needing garters to hold them in place; pantyhose, the all in one panty and hose; the slight control top pantyhose; the control top pantyhose for maximum tummy control; and, the total control pantyhose, with spandex in the panty and in the leg, for leg support as well.

Hosiery is manufactured in consumer-desired sheerness, from ultra sheer to opaque. The panty may be ultra sheer or opaque. Hosiery is manufactured as full-fashioned, which is knitted to the shape of the foot and leg, or in stretch nylon, which is tubular and takes on the shape of the leg of the wearer. Sizing runs as follows: short, average, tall, and Queen, and is based on the female's height and weight. Men's hose are best described as dress socks, worn with business or dress suits. They are full-fashioned and are calf or knee high. They are made of cotton, cotton blends, nylon, and fine wool.

HOT ITEMS Accessory or apparel items suddenly in great consumer demand. A fad. The demand usually cools off as suddenly as it began.

HOT PANTS *see* Shorts

HOUNDSTOOTH *see* Check

HOUSEDRESS Older terminology for day time dress worn by women when working in the home. Not fashion apparel.

HUARACHE (hə rä′ chē) Flat sandal with the upper made of woven strips of leather. Of Mexican and Spanish origin.

ICE DYE Azoic dyes used on cottons and some acetates, polyesters, and nylons. Known as ice dye because the reaction that produces the dyeing takes place at a lowered temperature. Colorfastness is good, but has tendency to crock.

IKAT (ee căt) Ancient and unusual process of resist printing. Warp yarns on a loom are covered with a resist material such as wax or clay, in areas of the design that the weaver does not desire the dye to absorb. The warp yarns are then dyed, the resist is removed, and the filling yarns are woven in. Finished fabric has shimmering, and indistinct, beautiful pattern.

I.L.G.W.U. Stands for International Ladies Garment Workers Union. Formed in 1900. The Triangle Shirt Factory fire of 1911 led to more protective laws for garment workers. All apparel made by members of this union have the union label sewn to an inside seam for identification purposes.

IMPULSE ITEMS Customer buys a nonplanned item. Accessories tend to be an impulse purchase, as well as items placed on or near the cash register and wrap counter.

INDIGO Blue dye obtained from India or produced synthetically.

INFLATION Sharp rise of prices due to an abnormal increase in available currency and credit, relative to available goods. Leads to a decline in the purchasing power of money.

INNERWEAR All areas of intimate apparel.

INORGANIC FIBERS Sometimes called mineral fibers. Lack the element carbon. Consists of: asbestos, from mineral deposits; glass, from silica sand and limestone; and metallic, such as gold, silver, stainless steel, and aluminum.

INSEAM Industry measurement of men's inner pant leg seam from the crotch to hem. Determines leg length for retail sale.

INSPIRATION, DESIGNERS Designers find sources of inspiration for their new collections from a variety of places and people. Famous individuals with a style or look, (Garbo, Monroe, Hepburn); from current events or countries in the world with a "look," (Scottish); from decades or centuries with a "look;" (medieval, the 1940's); from street fashions, especially of youth, (London); from flowers and colors; from a piece of artwork; famous movie or television personalities, (Madonna, Jacksons); sports events of today or the past, (horseback riding); or the distinctive dress of other cultures, (Russian, African). They interpret it in their own distinctive style.

INTARSIA Retail term for sweaters with geometric designs.

INTERFACING Manufacturer's term for fabric placed between two layers of fashion fabric for added body. Typically used in collars, lapels, cuffs, and buttoned openings.

INTERLOCK KNIT Knit fabric produced on a special machine, with a slight rib structure. Slightly heavier than a single knit and more stable in width.

INTIMATE APPAREL Fashion industry term for women's lingerie, foundations, and loungewear.

INVISIBLE ZIPPER *see* Zippers

IRISH KNIT Large, cable stitch knit sweater. Also called *Fisherman's*

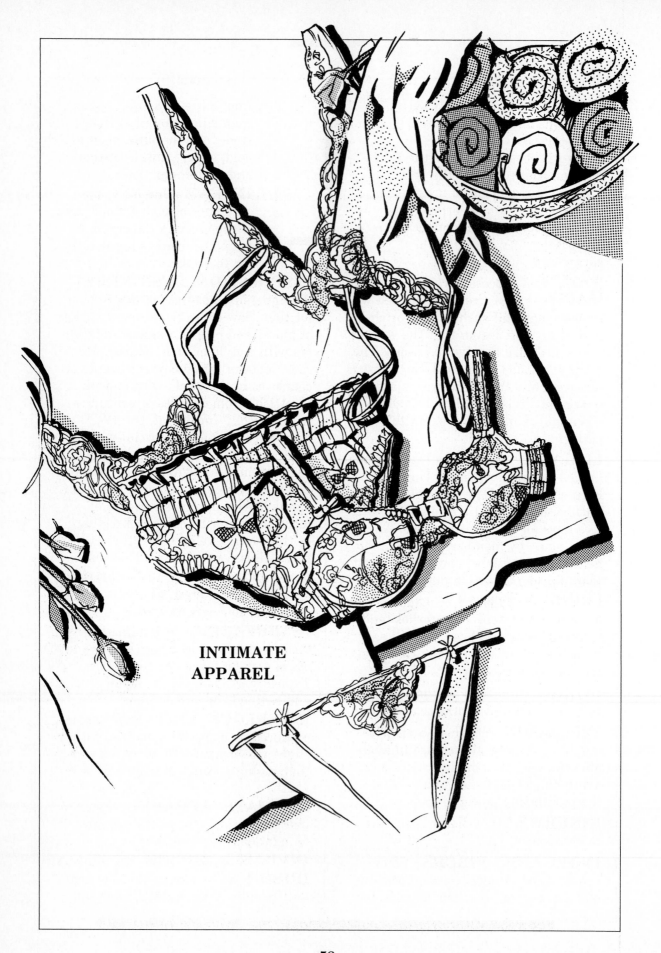

INTIMATE
APPAREL

knit. Originally hand knit and imported from Ireland. Most are now manufactured.

IRISH LINEN Fine linen fabric from flax plant, grown and processed in Ireland.

IRREGULARS Items of merchandise having defects affecting the appearance, not wear. Labeled and sold at a lesser price.

IVORY From the tusk of an elephant. Hard, smooth, yellow-white color. Carved into fans, combs, and jewelry. Elephants have been slaughtered for their tusks and are now protected by countries in Africa. Ivory look-a-likes are made of plastic.

IVY LEAGUE LOOK Classic look made popular in the 1940's and 1950's by male students from prestigious universities with ivy towers and such, primarily of the eastern United States. Narrow suit jacket, trousers and buttoned-down shirt, diagonal stripe tie.

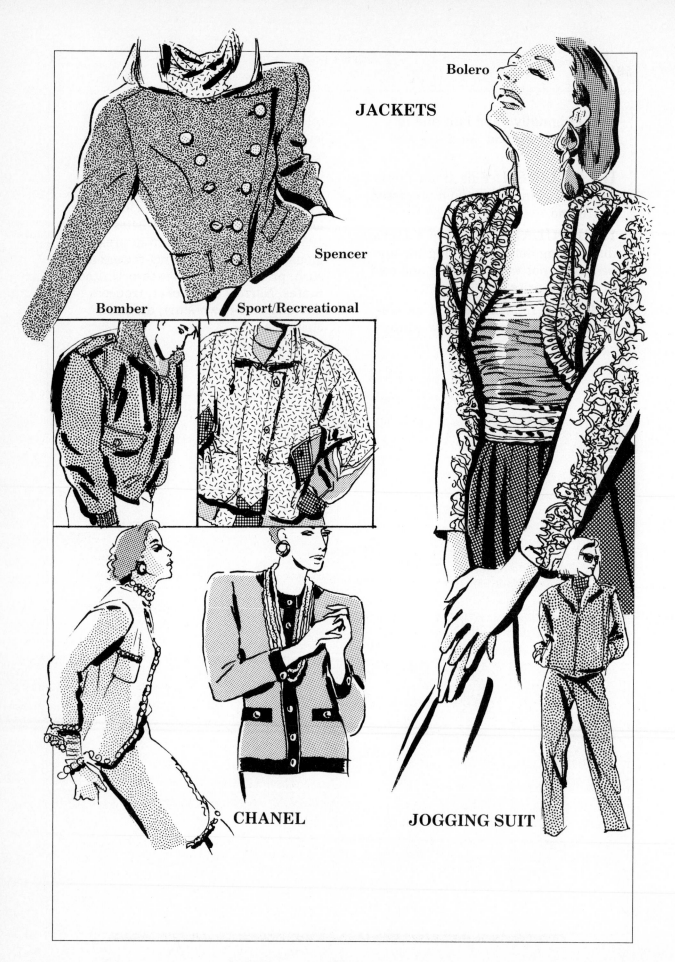

JACKETS

Bolero

Spencer

Bomber

Sport/Recreational

CHANEL

JOGGING SUIT

60

JABOT (zh/a bō′) Cascade of ruffles down the front of blouses, sometimes decorative and with lace trims. Attached or detachable. Of French origin.

JACKET A short coat worn by men or women. May be single-breasted, double-breasted, zippered, or wrapped. Dressy, casual, or functional (for warmth or protection from weather) depending upon design and fabrics used.

Battle/Bomber/Eisenhower Military-type blouson jacket made famous by a World War II general. Widely reproduced in leather, denims, and many other fabrications. *see* Eisenhower.

Blazer *see* Blazer

Bolero Short, waist length rounded front jacket, usually without a closure or collar. Sleeveless or with sleeves. Beginning with their use by men in early Crete, boleros have been worn by men and women throughout the centuries. Most commonly seen as a part of a men's Spanish bullfighter's costume.

Chanel Simple, short, collarless, straight-lined, braid-trimmed jacket, with or without center button closure. Made famous by Coco Chanel.

Dinner Dressy men's jacket, less formal than the tuxedo. Began in 1900 for formalwear. In the 1950's, used for summer formalwear. Replaced by the tuxedo in winter.

Eton Jacket style adapted in England from a jacket worn at Eton College. A little boy's straight jacket.

Nehru Adapted from a style worn by Prime Minister Nehru of India in the 1950's. A straight, single-breasted, mandarin collar, button to neck men's jacket.

Recreational Any type of short or hip-length jacket, used for protection from weather during, or after, a recreational sport such as golf, skiing, football, tennis, hiking, and more.

Spencer Originally worn by men who copied the look of a jacket worn by Lord Spencer of England in the 1800's. Short, fitted jacket now worn by women.

Tuxedo Jacket of the two or three piece formalwear suit. Style of jacket varies from waist length, suit length, to a jacket with tails. May be shawl collared, single- or double-breasted. Colors vary with the styles of the time: white, colored, grey, or black. *see* Suits, formal.

Unconstructed Unfitted jacket of many fabrications, usually unlined. More casual use.

JACQUARD Complex loom, descended from the oriental draw loom. Perfected in 1805 by Joseph Jacquard. The loom has the ability to produce complex, reversible patterns through punched and coded cards that control each yarn separately. Of French origin.

Knit Wide variety of patterned fabrics produced on weft knit machine including sweater knits with argyle, Fair Aisle, and intarsia patterns.

Woven Best known jacquard woven patterns include brocade and damask, and many dress/blouse fabrics.

JAPANESE American styles adapted from the Japanese culture and costume, such as kimonos, sandals, and parasols.

JEANS Popular, durable indigo-colored fabric of warp face twill weave made into pants. First made into tents in 1849 by Levi Straus for California gold miners. Subsequently made into a durable workpant for gold miners and others. Acceptance of jeans as a fashion pant began in the 1960's, and grew stronger in the 1970's and 1980's. Jeans fashions spread among young people of all economic backgrounds and countries and moved up the age scale. Made into pantsuits, skirts, and jackets, and embellished with designs. Eventually produced in different colors. Also sandwashed and acid distressed to produce even more varied fashion sportswear.

JERSEY KNIT Single knit fabric, made with machines having one needlebed and one set of needles. Fabric made of various fibers, cotton being predominant. Referred to as *jersey* by the retail market. Originally a woolen sweater worn by fishermen from the Isle of Jersey. Of English origin.

JESTER Costume of a buffoon in the medieval courts. Consisting of a short jacket (doublet), tights, peaked cap, bells, and multicolored throughout.

JEWEL Ornament of precious metal or gem worn as adornment.

JEWEL NECKLINE *see* Neckline

JEWELRY Jewels, collectively, such as bracelets, necklaces, earrings, pins, and rings.

JOBBER The middleman who buys from the manufacturer and sells to the retailers.

JOCKEY Costume of a professional racehorse rider. The colors used are from the one who owns the stable of horses. Costume consists of shirt, pants, jacket, and cap.

JODHPURS *see* Pants

JOGGING/RUNNING SUIT Exercise running apparel of the 1980's-1990's. Consists of shorts and a T or tank top, or full-length coordinated jacket and sweat pant. Recreation apparel also worn as casualwear.

JUMPER Sleeveless dress worn over a blouse, shirt, or sweater. Often an item of little girls apparel.

JUMPSUIT Worksuit worn to protect clothing, from 1900's. In the late 1960's, developed as fashion sportswear, eveningwear, and recreational wear for skiing.

JUNIOR SIZING Size range of women's apparel with shorter neck to waist and mature figure, sizes 3–15. Sometimes considered younger, more trendy designs.

JUTE Bast fiber from the stem of the jute plant. Fine, soft, lustrous fiber. Major use is in the making of burlap. Limited use in accessories such as belts.

KAPOK Hair fiber grown like cotton in a seed pod on the kapok tree. Dried fiber easily separated from seeds. Kapok is brittle, cannot be spun into yarns. Used as stuffing or filling.

KARAKUL Curled, wiry hair fiber from Karakul sheep. Woven fabric resembling this, used as furlike trim on coats.

KARAT (kar′ ət) "K" is the symbol of karat. Refers to the proportion of gold, measured in twenty-fourths of an item. Twenty-four karat is 24K, 100% gold. Other common gold proportions, worldwide, are 22K, 18K, 14K, and 10K. The law states that the amount of gold must be stamped on an item. Gold is alloyed with copper, silver, or nickel, to achieve lower cost and various colors.

KERCHIEF 1. A woman's square cloth, often worn as a head covering. 2. A handkerchief.

KEYHOLE *see* Neckline

KHAKI (kak′ ē) 1. A color ranging from olive-brown to a light yellowish-brown. 2. Durable cloth of this color. 3. Uniforms of this cloth.

KID Young goat. Leather made from the skin of a young goat.

KILT Knee-length, fully pleated, wrap skirt of tartan wool worn by men of the Scottish Highlands. Each Scottish clan has its distinctive colored tartan (plaid). Also worn by women and children.

KIP Animal skins weighing 15 to 25 pounds.

KNEE BREECHES Shorter, full pants, cuffed just below the knees.

KNICKERS/KNICKERBOCKERS *see* Pants

KNIT/KNITTING Construction of outerwear, fabrics, hosiery, and underwear by interlocking loops of yarn. In late 1500's, knitting from machine had been invented by William Lee, allowing knits that were formerly handmade to now be made mechanically. Knits are interlocking loops of yarn done horizontally (weft knit) or vertically (warp knit).

KNITTED APPAREL Knitted hosiery and sweaters are made on full-fashioned machines, by adding or decreasing knit stitches until the desired shape is obtained. *Fashion marks* are visible areas where stitches have been dropped or added. Apparel knitted as such is more stable. Knit shirts are made full-fashioned or from knitted fabric. The knit T (tee) is the most popular, with sleeves and/or pockets. The rugby is a wide striped, colored T; the Henley is a placket front T; and the polo shirt has a collar and short sleeves.

KNITTING, CONSTRUCTION
There are two types of knits—weft and warp. The weft knits include:
Double knit On rib machine with twice the yarn. Fabric has greater durability, less stretch.
High pile fabric Plain knit with heavy yarn for the background and addition of a carded sliver for the pile.
Interlock Special machine creates rib structure, more stable.
Jersey or single knit One set of needles and one needlebed. Uses: sweater, T shirts, other.
Knitted terry or velour Two yarns used simultaneously on jersey machine. As terry is knitted, face yarn is pulled out to produce loops. Velour is constructed the same, and then sheared to produce a soft surface.

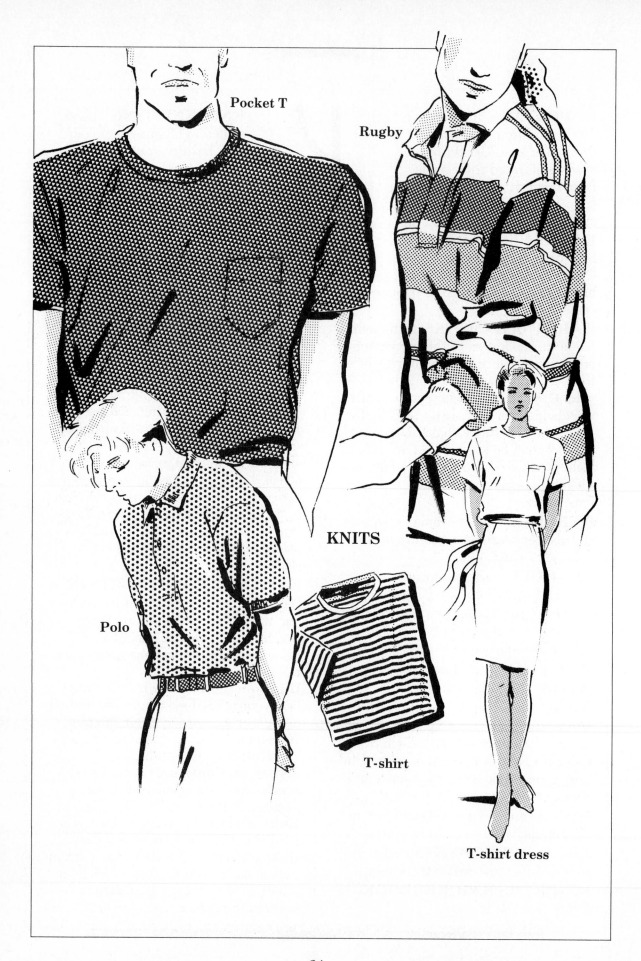

Pocket T

Rugby

Polo

KNITS

T-shirt

T-shirt dress

64

Purl Machines with two needlebeds. Adds decorative texture.

Rib knit On rib machine with alternating stitches to achieve fabric with great stretch.

The warp knits include:

Raschel Specialized machine. Produces laces to heavy fabrics—swimsuits and netting to carpets.

Tricot (trē′ kō) Using tricot machines. High volume is produced. Wide use in lingerie, sleepwear.

KNITS, PERFORMANCE Knit apparel is comfortable since it moves with the body, is easily cared for, and does not wrinkle. Problems can be shrinkage, stretching, and snagging—breaking of a knit loop, causing a "run" or a hole.

KNOCKOFF Fashion industry term referring to copying an item, usually at a lower price. There is no United States law against knockoff apparel or accessories. There are knockoff designers, knockoff manufacturers, and knockoff retailers.

KOHL Black preparation used in ancient days as eye makeup. The look was revived in the 1970's, using noncontaminating substances.

LABEL Means of identification. 1. Piece of cloth, stitched at the back neck or back waist of a garment, identifying manufacturer. 2. Care label for apparel as mandated by the Federal Trade Commission, to be sewn in a visible place on apparel, naming fiber content(s), recommended care procedures, and country of origin. 3. Fur regulations label the English name of animal, country of origin, type of processing used including dyeing, and if paws or tails were used. 4. Cosmetic labeling requires, for all except fragrances, that ingredients be listed on the container or package in order of predominance.

LABEL, PRIVATE Manufacturer which produces merchandise to certain specifications, under a special name for retail stores. The opposite of "branded" merchandise.

LACE Delicate weblike fabric. Design is created by threads alone. Handmade until the lace machine was invented by John Leaver in the early 1800's. Knitted lace is made on the Raschel machine. The Schiffli machine produces a lacelike embroidered fabric—not true lace. Early handmade laces took on the names of the towns producing their certain pattern. Two main types of lace making are: bobbin or pillow lace, using knotted, twisted threads (related to netting and knotting) and needlepoint lace (related to embroidery). Many laces are produced, well-known ones include:

Alençon (ə len' sən) Needlepoint lace with sheer net background and solid design outlined in cord. Of French origin.

Battenberg Application of linen Battenberg tape to design and to connect with decorative stitches.

Belgium Pillow lace from areas of Belguim.

Chantilly Fine lace in which designs are outlined in heavy thread. Of French origin.

Cluny Heavier bobbin lace in designs of a wheel or other design. Of French origin.

Milanese Bobbin lace made by joining fine mesh with tapes to form patterns such as flowers and figures. Of Italian origin.

Rose point Needlepoint lace from Venice. Of Italian origin.

Valenciennes Flat bobbin lace, used for edgings. Of French origin.

LAMBSKIN Leather made from the skin of a young sheep—lamb.

LAMBSWOOL Fine wool from first shearing of a lamb. *see* Wool.

LAMÉ (la mā') Metallic fabric with metallic fiber, used as warp or filling yarns.

LAMINATED Outer fabric is joined to a material such as polyurethane foam by the use of an adhesive.

LAPEL Extension of the garment that is sewn to the collar and folds back over the chest area. Typical in jackets and coats and also in some blouses and dresses. Notched lapel is the most classic. Higher fashion menswear lapels are semi or peaked, with a sharply pointed extension.

LAPIDARY Person who works at cutting and polishing gems.

LARGE Denotes size large. Symbol "L" in women's and menswear when sizing is not labeled in numbers. Is a more approximate sizing method.

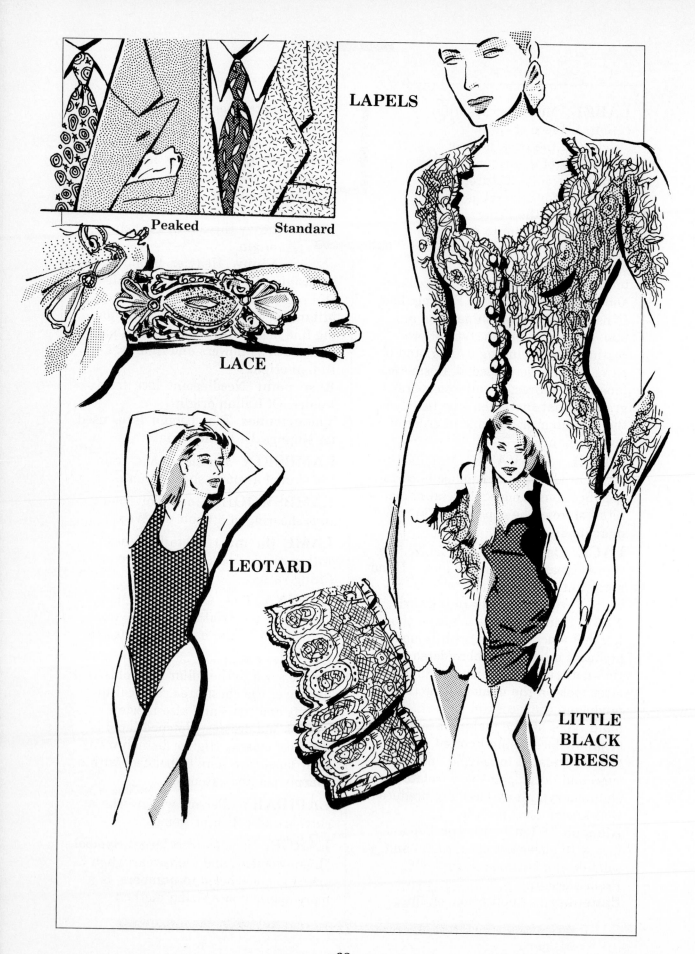

LAPELS

Peaked   Standard

LACE

LEOTARD

LITTLE
BLACK
DRESS

68

LAST Molded shape of human foot from which shoes are designed and manufactured.

LASTEX® Trademark for a yarn with a core of elastic rubber covered with cotton or other fiber and used in apparel for stretch areas.

LAVALIERE (lav′ a lir′) Pendant worn on a chain around the neck. Of French origin.

LAVENDER Pale purple color.

LAWN Fine, sheer crisp-finish plain weave cotton or other fiber.

LAYETTE Collection of apparel and nonclothing items needed for a newborn baby. Includes undershirts, diapers, nightgowns, receiving blankets, socks or bootees, toys, and feeding items.

LEAF FIBERS Limited use in fashion. Pina cloth, from the pineapple plant is used to make sheer, lustrous shirts. Of Philippine origin.

LEASED DEPARTMENT A department within a store that is leased and operated by another company and pays a percentage of sales to the store as rent. The outside company owns the stock, merchandises and staffs the department, and runs the department as an overall part of the store. Typical leased departments are fine jewelry, shoes, furs, beauty salon, and other small service areas.

LEATHERS Tanned hide of an animal, reptile, marine life, or bird, usually with hair removed. Animals used for leather include: cow, sheep, pig, calf, kid, and deer; marine life such as eel; and other creatures such as snake, alligator, or ostrich. Finishes include: napping to raise hair fibers for a soft finish product termed suede; glazing for a shiny finish; polyurethane coating to produce glossy patent leather; boarding to produce soft creased leather; and embossing, a stamped pattern of another animal to produce an 'animal-like' effect. Hides are split—cut horizontally. The top layer is the finest and labeled top grain. Other layers are termed "splits," and the layer nearest the flesh is of the least quality. Leathers are used for apparel—tops, pants, jackets, coats, and many accessory items such as handbags, belts, shoes, small leather items, and some hats and jewelry.

LEG WARMERS Knitted covering for legs, originally worn by ballet dancers. A fashion item for aerobics, dancers, and others.

LEISURE SUIT Mens double knit suit of the 1960's.

LENGTH Defined lower edge of a garment. Jacket lengths include waist, hip, and thigh length; skirts include mini, above and below knee, calf, ankle, and full or floor length; coats include thigh, calf/full, and floor lengths; sleeves include cap, short, three-quarter, and full lengths. Current fashion includes many length options available.

LENO Open, gauzelike fabric, constructed by leno attachment that crosses lapped yarns while a filling yarn passes through.

LEOTARD Snug fitting, elastic one-piece garment worn for dancing or exercising. Now in fashion colors and designs. Often worn over fashion colored tights (leg covers). Unitard is a one-piece neck to ankle garment, combining leotard and tights.

LET-OUT Complex cutting of smaller fur skins into small strips to be resewn. Used to maintain the natural look of the animal in a full size garment.

LETTICE EDGING Small, ruffled edging on dress or lingerie.

LICENSING Contract where firms manufacture and market apparel or accessory items in the name of the designer, popular sports or entertainment individual, and others. Licensor is then paid a percentage of sales. In 1950, Christian Dior was the first designer to license his name. The advantage of licensing is that merchandise is generally more saleable due to the name recognition.

LINE Group of new designs for a season. Collection—top designer's line for the new season.

LINE-FOR-LINE COPY Original design is mass-produced in similar, but less costly fabric and in standardized sizes.

LINEN Oldest known fiber, from the stem of the flax plant. Bast fiber is produced by soaking (retting process) the stems, causing them to break down allowing the woody stem to separate from the inner fiber. Linen is 5 to 20 inches long, strong and stable, absorbent, lacks elasticity, resists insects, and may mildew. Can be woven sheer to very coarse. Major disadvantage is high price of apparel and wrinkling.

LINGERIE Category of women's undergarments: slips, camisoles, panties, sleepwear, nightgowns, and pajamas.

LINING Fabric used to finish garment insides, hide seams, retain shape, make opaque, or enhance general appearance and quality. Typical use in coats, jacket, and skirts. Also in sheer or better dresses, and better pants.

LIPSTICK Cosmetic item used to color lips.

LITTLE BLACK DRESS Simple black dress that cycles through fashion. Worn with accessories.

LLAMA Camel-like, domesticated animal of the Andes Mountains. Lustrous brown or black hair fiber, used for apparel.

LOOK Accessories and apparel combined, which carry out a general theme or look. Certain looks are more cyclical, such as ethnic, nautical, western, or romantic. Some looks have come from movies or television influences, such as the movie *Annie Hall* and the subsequent layered look. The prairie look, preppie look from Ivy League college students, safari, punk, and other looks inspired by movies or culture.

LOOM Piece of machinery from small hand variety to huge complex automated looms. Interlaces yarns at right angles and weaves fabric. Warp are lengthwise yarns and fillings are horizontal yarns.

LOOP *see* Closure

LOUIS HEEL *see* Heels

LOUNGEWEAR Category of apparel, including robes to caftans, and at-home clothing.

LUREX® Decorative metallic appearance yarn made of a layer of aluminum between two layers of polyester film, protected by a clear or colored resin coating.

LYCRA® DuPont trademark name for spandex fiber.

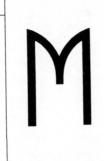

MACKINAW Short, double-breasted, heavy woolen coat, usually plaid.

MACKINTOSH Any raincoat.

MACRAME Openwork, made by use of looping and a variety of ornamental knotting. Decoration on clothing and wall hangings.

MADDER Use of root of madder plant to obtain rich red dye.

MADEIRA Type of embroidery.

MADRAS Cotton cloth, usually plaids or checks, originated in Madras, India.

MAGAZINES, FASHION Began with *Godey's Lady's Book*, both fashion and informational, begun 150 years ago. Current fashion magazines include *Vogue, Young Miss, Harper's Bazaar, Mademoiselle, Mirabelle, Glamour*, and *Elle*. All are both fashion and informational, with articles of current interest to women. *Gentlemen's Quarterly* is exclusively men's fashions and articles of current interest.

MALTESE CROSS Cross in the form of four arrowheads, smaller toward the center. Used as ornamental jeweled pins.

MANDARIN *see* Collars.

MAN-MADE FIBER Fibers created through chemical means, with qualities to make them useful in textiles. The synthetic polymers are converted to liquid form, extruded through a spinneret as a filament yarn. Nylon, polyester, acrylic, modacrylic, and spandex are petroleum-based man-made fibers used for fashion apparel and accessories. Man-made cellulosic fibers include rayon, acetate, and triacetate.

MANNEQUIN/MANIKIN Model of the human body used to display fashion apparel and accessories.

MANTILLA (man ti′ ə) Large lace scarf, usually black or white, worn over head and shoulders. (Sp).

MANUFACTURER Company that makes or processes an item into a finished product. In fashion industry there are manufacturers of fabrics, apparel, and accessories.

MARCASITE Silverlike metal (iron pyrite) polished and used for jewelry.

MARKDOWN Price lowered less than original retail price.

MARKET 1. Target customers. 2. Place where buyers of apparel and accessories meet manufacturer's representatives to view and order merchandise. 3. Business of buying and selling merchandise.

MARKET CENTER Main area of a nation. The New York market is the center of the fashion industry with all major designers and manufacturers represented. Next in importance are the Los Angeles market and Dallas market. Regional markets primarily handle the business of an area of the country, with limited numbers of designers and representatives.

MARKETING Buying and selling of merchandise, including plan, pricing, and distributing of merchandise for sale to customers.

MARKET WEEK Designated weeks in a year highlighting the new lines for a season: womenswear, childrens, menswear, and accesssories. Buyers view and order merchandise for retail stores from the sales reps of the manufacturers.

MARKUP Difference between wholesale cost and retail price of merchandise.

MAROON Dark, reddish-brown to purplish-red color.

MART Building with showrooms of sample garments of merchandise for that selling season.

MASS FASHION Fashions that are widely accepted and worn by most people.

MATELASSE (mat′ lə sā′) Luxurious designed, padded fabric, made with four sets of yarns. Of French origin.

MATERNITY Clothing made especially to fit women expecting a baby.

MATTE (mat) Dull finish on metals or fabric.

MAUVE (môv) Greyed, reddish-purple color.

MAXI Ankle or floor length coat or skirt, from the 1960's.

MEDIUM Denotes size medium. Symbol "M" in womens and menswear, when sizing is not labeled in numbers. Is a more approximate sizing method.

MELTON Heavy, durable wool fabric for coating. Of English origin.

MERCERIZATION Process of treating cotton fabric, under tension to avoid shrinkage, with caustic soda to increase luster. Also strengthens fabric and increases dyeability.

MERCHANDISE ASSORTMENT Collection of various types of related merchandise.

MERCHANDISING Planning, buying, and selling of fashion apparel and accessories.

MERINO Breed of sheep that produces the most valuable and finest quality wool.

METALLIC FIBERS/YARN Manufacture of fiber composed of metal, plastic-coated metal, metal-coated plastic, or a core completely covered by metal.

METALS, JEWELRY Precious metals are gold, silver, and platinum. Base metals are copper, brass, nickel, iron, pewter, and others. Alloy is a combination of metals.

Gold Metal with properties of ductile; can be drawn into fine threadlike wire; malleable, hammered thin; indestructible. Use of alloyed gold produces some color differences: gold and copper, pinkish color; gold and silver, light green color; gold with copper, zinc, or nickel, white gold. Most American jewelry is 14K gold.

Silver The metal of royalty. Properties are ductile, malleable, tarnishes, and corrodes. Pure silver is 99.9 percent silver. Sterling silver is 92.5 percent pure silver alloyed with 7.5 percent copper. Quality mark is required.

Platinum Rarest, hardest of metals. Silverlike color. Does not oxidize or tarnish. Quality mark required. Used only in the last three centuries when tools were invented to work with it. Ductile and malleable.

Base metals Used alone or in alloys with precious metals. No quality mark required when used alone.

Electroplate Thin layer of precious metal is applied over base metal through process of water bath and electric current used for application of precious metal. Must be identified as such, for example, silverplate. Less expensive items produced.

MICRO Very short skirt or dress length, from the 1960's.

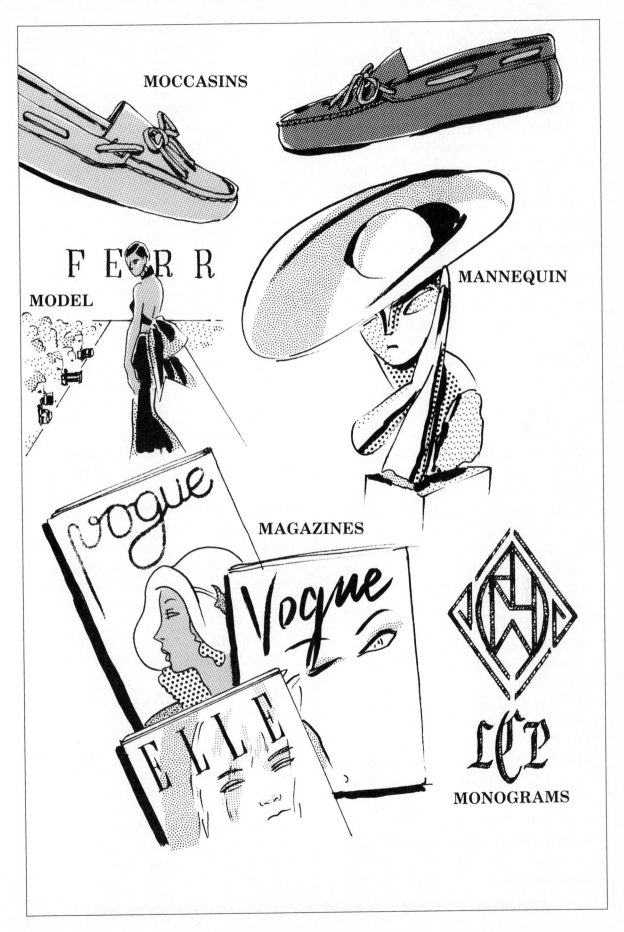

MOCCASINS

MODEL

F E R R

MANNEQUIN

MAGAZINES

MONOGRAMS

MIDDY Pertaining to a nautical top or blouse.

MIDI Longer skirt length, mid or below calf, from the 1970's.

MIDRIFF Part of the female body or clothing, or lack of clothing, in the area below the breasts to waist.

MILANESE *see* Lace

MILDEW Fungus or mold discoloration on damp fabric, particularly cotton and linen.

MILL END Short pieces of fabric at end of bolt. Usually sold at a discount.

MILLINER One who makes or sells women's hats.

MILLINERY Women's hats.

MINAUDIERE *see* Handbags

MINERAL FIBERS Classification of inorganic fibers such as asbestos and glass.

MINI Something smaller or shorter, such as a miniskirt.

MINK A large weasel animal known and used for its thick, luxurious fur pelt. Color range is white to deep, rich brown. *see also* Furs.

MISSES SIZE Size range includes even numbers, usually 4 to 16, for women 5'4" or over and average body proportion.

MITTEN Hand covering with one area for the thumb and remaining larger area for four fingers.

MOCCASIN Soft leather slipper or shoe, resembling those worn by American Indians.

MOCHA Light coffee color.

MODACRYLIC Man-made fiber of modified acrylic formula. Used in high pile, fleece, fake fur fabrics, wigs, hair pieces, and other apparel. Characteristics include fire retardant, good stability, light weight, and good insulating properties.

MODEL Person employed to display clothing and accessories by wearing them for fashion shows, advertising, and publicity.

MOHAIR Hair fiber from angora goat, sheared for hair removal. Similar characteristics to sheep's wool except for high luster and slippery, smooth surface. Current use in men's and women's suiting. Quality and costs are high.

MOIRÉ (mwä rā′) Fabric with watery appearance, obtained by process of placing one length of fabric over the other and applying pressure. A roller method can also be used. Flattened fabric areas reflect light differently to achieve moiré look. Of French origin.

MONK'S CLOTH Coarse, basket weave fabric with four warp and four filling yarns.

MONOFILAMENT Extrusion of one filament of yarn. Limited to use in very sheer hosiery. Most yarns are multifilament.

MONOGRAM Design sewn on garment composed of one or more letters. Usually one's initials.

MOTHER-OF-PEARL Internal, pearly layer of certain mollusk shells. Used for jewelry and buttons.

MUFF Tubular accessory item with open ends for one's hands to be placed for warmth. Often of fur or special fabrics.

MULTIFILAMENT YARNS Yarn having more than one filament, can be twisted together tightly or loosely.

MUSK Secretion from gland of male musk deer, otter, or civet. Used in making certain fragrances.

MUSLIN Plain weave cotton, of various qualities, typically unbleached and tannish in color.

MUUMUU Long, loose colorful dress, hangs free from shoulders. Of Hawaiian origin.

MYLAR Metallic yarn of a layer of aluminum sandwiched between two layers of clear or colored polyester film.

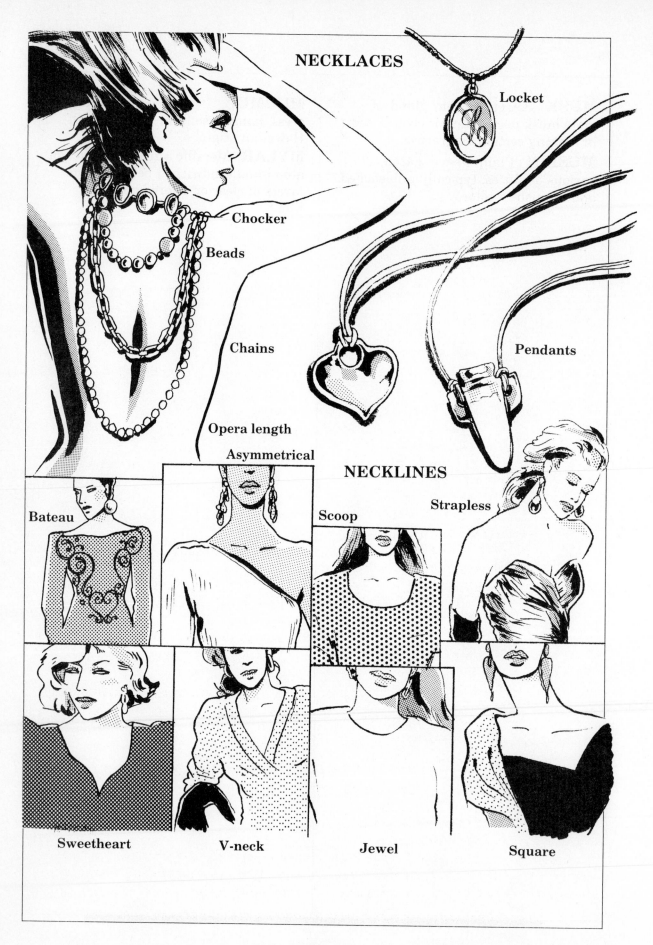

NECKLACES

Locket

Chocker

Beads

Chains

Pendants

Opera length

Asymmetrical

NECKLINES

Bateau

Scoop

Strapless

Sweetheart

V-neck

Jewel

Square

NAP/NAPPING Fiber ends are brushed up on surface of fabric for a soft look and feel. Flannel and brushed denim are examples.

NATURAL FIBERS Any fiber present in or produced by nature; of animal, vegetable, or mineral source. Two main categories: cellulose (plant), cotton and linen; and protein, wool and other hair, and silk.

NAUTICAL Pertaining to the personnel and ships of the navy. In fashion, many designs are from nautical source, including the nautical "look": middy collar, sailor pant and cap, pea jacket, and nautical colors of blue and white.

NECKLACES Have been in evidence since earliest civilization. First seen as massive gold and semiprecious collars or ornate pendants on ancient Egyptians. Necklaces of Greek women were of gold, in animal forms, pendants, stone cameos, and small vials with scents hanging as pendants on gold chains. Roman necklaces were massive in size and contained precious gems, as well as the wearing of ropes of pearls.

In the Baroque era, necklaces were a simple, single strand of pearls. Jewelry of the 1700's in France was elegant chokers of precious stones, or no necklace to better expose the white skin of women. After the French Revolution, a simple ribbon was worn at base of neck. Then came a period of no necklace with bare décolletage in fashion.

With the high necklines of the 1900's, women wore pearl necklaces. Great ropes of glass beads and imitation pearls, introduced by Chanel, were worn in the 1920's. Costume jewelry has been worn and accepted since this time. The 1960's was a period of wearing gold chains, by both men and women. The hippies wore love beads of seeds and shells. Current styles include pearls, large faux or semiprecious beads and pendants.

Beads Various items, with two holes and threaded on a string. Items used include seeds, shells, glass, crystal, stones, pearls, and all semiprecious and precious stones, as well as plastic copies. Vary in length from base of neck to long, hanging length.

Bib Fuller necklace fitting close at neck and covering the front area of chest.

Chain Interlocking small to very large links of metal, silver, gold, or electroplated. May have stones or gems for added beauty. Many lengths.

Choker Necklace of two or more strands that fit from base of neck upward.

Collar Wider necklace, fitting like a collar.

Locket Gold or silver disk hangs on a chain, with opening for a picture or lock of hair.

Opera/rope Extremely long strand of beads, usually wound into two strands.

Pendant Chain with ornament hung at center front. Jeweled ornament, medallion, zodiac, cross, or other.

Squash Very large, ornate necklace covering most of wearer's chest, of turquoise and silver, in ornate design, originally made and worn by southwestern United States Indians.

Zodiac Sign from one's horoscope.

NECKLINE Line formed by the edge of the garment at the neck. Current styles include:

Asymmetric Any off-center design.

Bandeau Straight, strapless neckline created by band above breasts, exposing chest and shoulders in a straight line.

Bateau (ba tō)/boat High, straight line from shoulder to shoulder.

Built-up Neckline extends higher than base of neck.

Crew/jewel Round neckline, fits to body at base of neck. Crew, as in a sweater, and jewel, as in a blouse or dress.

Halter Front of garment is sleeveless and fabric wraps from underarm up and around back of neck, usually with a V front.

Keyhole High neckline with a teardrop hole in front, near neckline.

Off-the-shoulder/strapless May be bandeau look or strapless and shaped to body as in a bustier.

Peasant/gathered Neckline has cord or elastic to draw up fabric into gathers in a rounded neckline.

Scoop Any mid, low, or broad U-shaped curve.

Square Any variety of right angles, squares, or rectangles.

Surplice Wrap top which forms a V at center.

Sweetheart Series of side and lower front curves that meet in center.

V or VV Front, or back and front, VV's.

NECKTIE *see* Ties

NECKWEAR Category of scarves and ties.

NEEDLEPOINT Decorative needlework on canvas mesh with use of diagonal stitches.

NEGLIGEE (neg′ la zhā′) Women's loose, decorative dressing gown, usually coordinated with a nightgown.

NEON Colors so bright, they seem to glow.

NET Openwork fabric, created by looping and knotting. Made on bobbinet lace machine, also some raschel machines. Weights vary from very fine to heavy.

NEW LOOK Christian Dior introduced an entirely new, full skirted, soft look to fashion in 1947 after the end of World War II. It revolutionized fashion and thus acquired this name.

NIGHT CLOTHES Older term for nightwear.

NIGHTGOWN/NIGHTIE Loose gown of many lengths and styles, worn to bed by females. People of earlier civilizations often wore underwear to bed. Current styles vary from simple, unadorned with shoulder straps, sleeveless or with sleeves, short, to long lengths, in cotton, polyester, blends, and silk. Equally available are very decorative styles with lace, embroidery, and ribbon trim, most costly are of silk. Full-length cotton flannel nightgowns, complete with high neck and long sleeve is usually worn when additional warmth is required. Baby Doll nightgown was a very short, full nightie with matching panties, from the 1960's.

NONWOVEN FABRICS Other fabrication method, exclusive of woven and knits, includes: felt; polymer films, a coating on fabrics such as vinyl-coated for leatherlike fabric and Ultrasuede ®, created to look and feel like suede leather; net, macrame; lace, and crochet.

NOTCHED *see* Lapel

NOVELTY YARNS Yarns made to create certain decorative textural effect. Fancy yarns include:

Boucle (bōō klā′) Yarn forming irregular loops around a base yarn.

Chenille yarn Pile fabric is created by loose ends of fiber that fluff up on surface, a soft, caterpillar look.

Core-spun yarn One fiber is wrapped around another. Major use as a stretch yarn.

Flake Flock or seed yarns. Weak, loosely twisted yarn.

Nub yarns Yarn is twisted around base yarn to create a bump in varying areas.

Slub yarn Irregular, loose and tightly twisted to create effect.

Spiral yarn Two-ply yarns, one is heavier and twists around the other.

NYLON Man-made synthetic polyamide fiber. Du Pont Company pioneered the earliest nylon in the United States. Characteristics include: excellent strength, lightweight, elasticity, good stability, moderately absorbent, and quick drying. Easy care for consumer.

Builds up static electricity because it is a poor conductor of electricity, resists moths, mildew, but tendency to scavenge or grey-out if white nylon is washed with other colors. Degraded by long exposure to sun. Major importance is use as women's hosiery. Used in blends with natural fiber, especially wool, to add wrinkle resistance.

NYLONS General term for women's hosiery.

NYTRIL Man-made fiber used for soft clothing, not currently being produced in the United States.

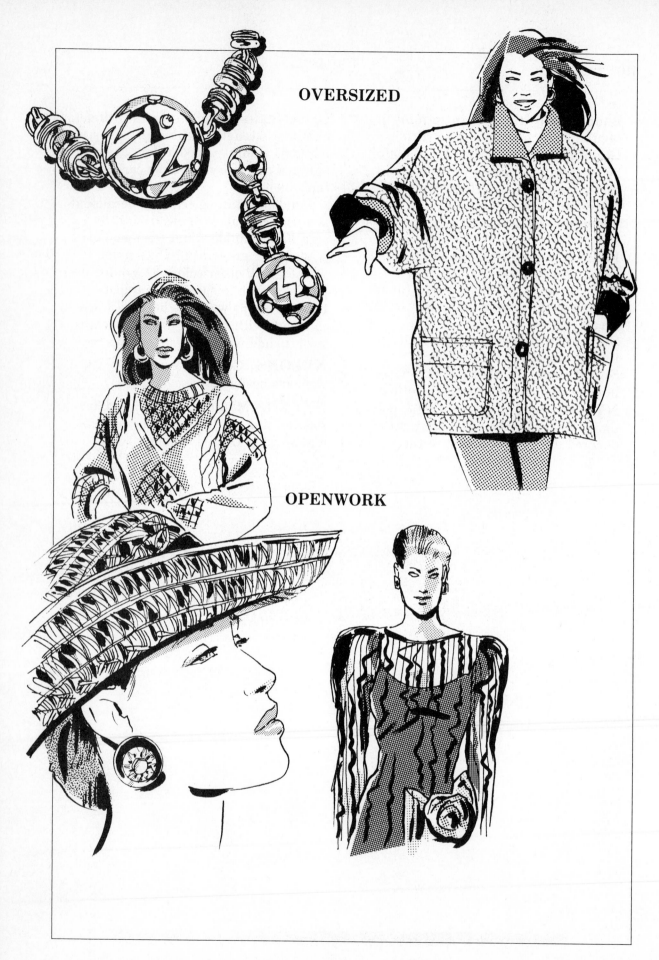

OVERSIZED

OPENWORK

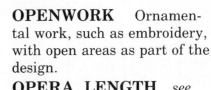

OBSOLESCENCE Old, past useful stage. In fashion cycle, it is the stage when clothing can no longer be sold at any price.

OFF-PRICE RETAIL Selling of brand name and/or designer label merchandise at lower than normal retail price. Much of the merchandise is from the past season, overruns in production, or irregulars. Some manufacturers have opened their own off-price stores, called factory outlets, and others sell to jobbers who then sell to an off-price retailer. A trend today is the emergence of off-price malls, with many off-price stores; from clothing and accessories to household items.

OFF-SHORE PRODUCTION American goods being produced in foreign, cheap-labor countries, with designs and specifications provided by United States management.

OFF-THE-SHOULDER *see* Necklines

ONYX *see* Gems

OPAL *see* Gems

OPAQUE (ō pāk′) Impenetrable by light. Opposite of transparent—totally visible.

OPENWORK Ornamental work, such as embroidery, with open areas as part of the design.

OPERA LENGTH *see* Necklaces

ORGANDY Sheer, crisp finish cotton fabric.

ORGANZA Similar to organdy, may have temporary or permanent crisp finish.

OSTRICH Fine, expensive leather with raised round markings from removal of feathers. Made from the skin of the African flightless bird.

OTTOMAN Fabric made of pronounced rib weave construction.

OUTRÉ (ōō trā′) To go to excess. Of French origin.

OVERALL *see* Pants

OVERSIZE Larger than needed size, but may be the fashion, as in oversize tops.

OXFORD CLOTH Firm, basket weave fabric of cotton or cotton blends, used for shirting. Plain-colored or with narrow-colored striped warp.

OXFORD SHOES Low heeled, laced shoe for men, women, or children. A classic men's oxford is the *wing tip*, with stitched wing pattern on toe of shoe and side perforation decor.

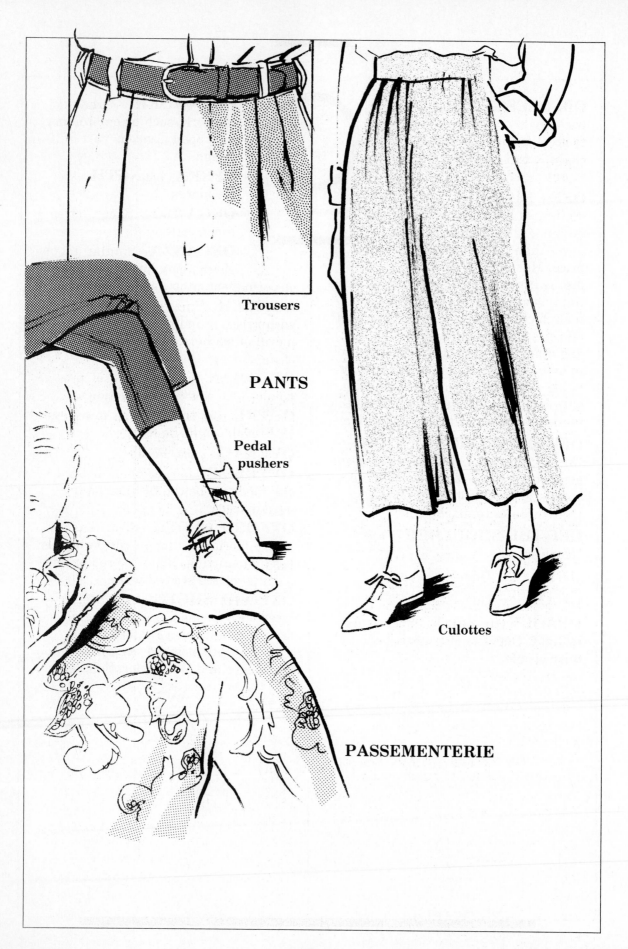

Trousers

PANTS

Pedal
pushers

Culottes

PASSEMENTERIE

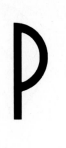

PADDING Additional material used between fabrics to give full or shaped look.

PADS, SHOULDER Triangles that fit over shoulder cap to heighten or extend silhouette. *see* Shoulder Pad.

PAGRI Also called pugree. East Indian turban. The use of designs and colors indicates prestige of wearer.

PAILLETTE (pà yet′) Shiny, flat round disk, larger than a sequin, sewn to garment for decorative trim.

PAISLEY Tear drop design on fabric or other material.

PAISLEY SHAWL Large fashion shawl of silk, with tear drop design, dates from early nineteenth century. Depending on size, the shawl was draped over head and shoulders.

PAJAMAS Sleeping or lounging two-piece garment for men, women, and children. Consisting of pant leg bottoms with attached or detached tops. Top is buttoned or slip-over-the-head type, with long or short sleeves. Beach pajamas were a sportswear innovation popular in the 1920's. Pajamas originated in India and were worn by men. From Hindu, pae (leg) and jamah (garment). Also called PJ's.

Attached Foot Design typical for small children, for additional warmth. Origination from Dr. Denton sleepers, from 1895.

Baby Doll/Teddies Design beginning in the 1960's, with decorative short top and panty. Also one piece.

Coat Style Design with a buttoned front.

Ski Design with cuffed wrists and ankles. Typical of childrenswear. From thermal underwear origination.

Slipover Design without buttoned front, to be put on over head.

PANACHE (pə nash′) Original use as plume of feathers on hat. Current use to note an individual with "style" and fashion individuality. Of French origin.

PANAMA HAT *see* Hats

PANAMA SUIT *see* Suits, Men

PANNE (pan) Fabric similar to velvet, with pile or raised surface that has been flattened for this desired look.

PANNIER (pan′ ē ər) A wire or framework to enlarge side of skirt at waist area. From 1700's.

PANNIER CRINOLINE An underskirt placed over pannier framework.

PANTALETTE Female underpants from 1800's. Long and full, and desirable to show below hem of dress.

PANTALOON 1. A type of male tight fitting trousers, from eighteenth century. 2. A term for women's underpants, from nineteenth century.

PANTIES Women's or girl's undergarment, covering the body below the waist. Shortened version of pantaloons. A full pantie has been popular since the 1920's. The longer version, also called bloomers, was the original creation of Amelia Jenks Bloomer, a nineteenth century feminist.

Bikini Panties beginning below navel, to top of leg. Introduced in the 1960's. A copy of the popular bathing suit. *see* Swimwear.

Brief Panties fit from the waist to beginning of leg.

French Cut Panties fit from waist to leg, with side hip cut high on the body.

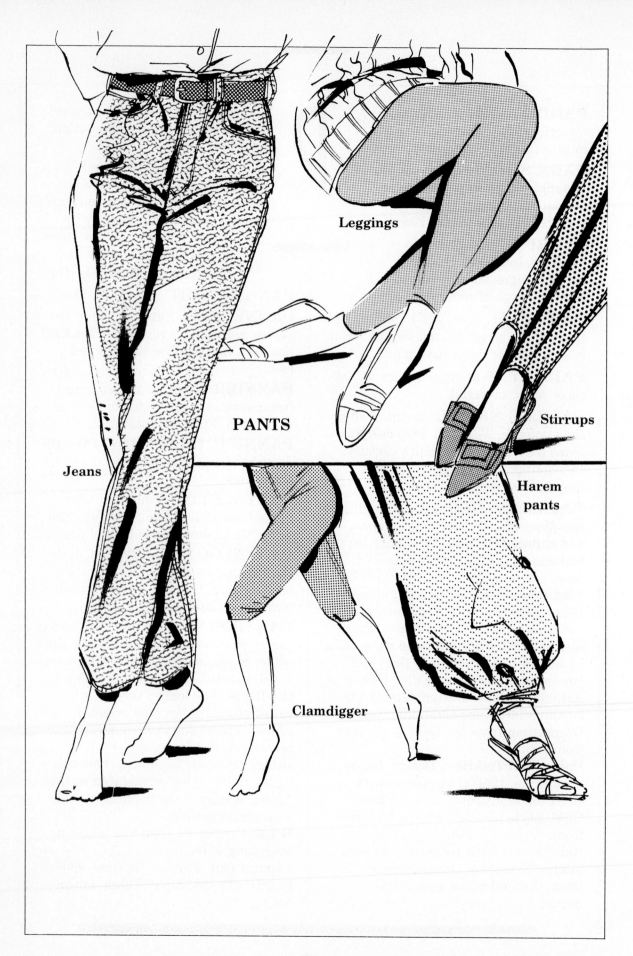

Leggings

Stirrups

PANTS

Jeans

Harem
pants

Clamdigger

Tap Full panties with side flare.

Tights Panties made of stretch fabric. May also include attached leg. Originally worn by dancers in the nineteenth century. *see also* Leotards; Pantyhose.

PANTS A garment for men, women, and children that encloses hips and legs. Either loose or fitted. Also called trousers or slacks. Originally worn by men, beginning in 1815. Women first wore a work pant during World War I when they replaced men in factory work. A lounging pant was popular in the 1920's. Pant suits for women were introduced in the 1960's.

Baggie Oversized pant.

Bell Bottoms/Flares Pants with varying fullness from knee to hem. From nautical look. A 1960's fashion pant.

Capri Women's tight fitting pants of the 1950's with narrow, tapered legs and ankle slits.

Clam Digger Calf length, tight fitting pant. A sportswear fashion of the 1950's.

Coveralls Originally a work pant for men with attached top and sleeves. Now also a fashion garment.

Culotte Women's flared, shortened pant, made to look like a skirt.

Fatigues/Dungarees Heavy work pant worn by United States military soldiers and sailors.

Gaucho Women's calf-length, wide pant, of Spanish origin.

Harem Women's pant, fully gathered into waist and ankle areas. Origin from Near East.

Hip Huggers Pant from 1960's that begins below typical waist area.

Hot Pants A popular short pant of the 1960's. *see also* Shorts.

Jeans/Levis/Dungarees Work pant made of denim, originally worn by sailors. Levi Co. trademark for a pant made for gold miners in California. Now a popular fashion pant. *see also* Jeans.

Jodhpurs/Riding Breeches Men or women's fashion horse riding pant with side fullness and tight fit from knee to ankle. Often with leather inner leg patches.

Jumpsuits Fashion pant with attached top and bottoms.

Knickers/Breeches/Knickerbockers/ Plus Fours Pant with full cut leg and fullness, sewn to knee or calf band.

Leggings Knit pantlike tights of heavier yarns or of lace, that fit the contour of leg.

Leiderhosen Short pant with suspenders and made of suede. From German origin.

Overalls/Bib Tops Traditional work pant with bib top and suspenders over shoulder and back. Also a style of ski pant.

Palazzo Women's long, wide leg, flared pant, first popular in the 1960's as evening wear.

Pedal Pushers Straight leg women's pant, shortened to calf length, often with cuffs. Popular in the 1950's.

Sailor/Bell Bottoms Traditional pant worn by members of the United States Navy, with button front closing and flared leg.

Ski Pant used for skiing. Two main types: 1. Regular pant or bib top with thermal padding for warmth. 2. Heavyweight stretch fabric pant with band under foot to anchor pant in place.

Stirrup Tight fitting pant with anchor band under foot.

Stovepipe/Cigarette Pant with narrow leg, originally worn by men in the 1800's.

Sweat Loose pant of fleece, typically used for recreational sports and now a

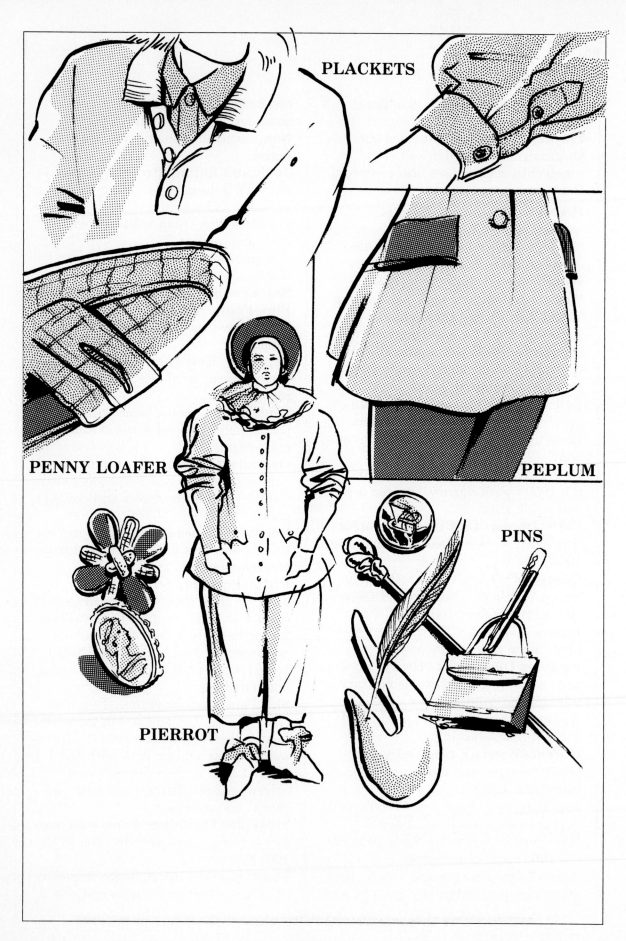

PLACKETS

PEPLUM

PENNY LOAFER

PINS

PIERROT

fashion pant. Often coordinated with a matching top.

Tailored/Trousers Pants with a classic look, with or without waist tucks. Fits to body with a straight leg. Optional cuffs.

PANTYHOSE All-in-one pantie and hose with attached foot. Toe and/or heel reinforcement, or sandlefoot, without reinforcement. Main types: sheer to opaque, with density differences from transparent to non-see-through; control top, with elastic in pantie to control fullness as in a lightweight girdle; and support hose, has added elastic in leg for additional support.

PARACHUTE CLOTH Lightweight fabric of nylon, similar to fabric used to make parachutes.

PARASOL Umbrella, often decorative, to protect from sun. Made of fabric or paper. Early Egyptian and Oriental origin.

PARKA Hooded jacket, usually made with padding or down inner layer, for warmth.

PASSEMENTERIE (pas men′ trē) Trimmings on garments for decoration. Use of beads, braids, ribbons, sequins, and others. From nineteenth century.

PATCH *see* Pocket

PATCHWORK Squares of various fabrics sewn together to form a fabric or applied decoration.

PATENT LEATHER *see* Leathers

PEA COAT/JACKET *see* Coats

PEARL *see* Gemstones

PEARL BUTTON Round, pearl-like button, usually of plastic or mother-of-pearl base.

PEASANT BLOUSE/SKIRT/

DRESS Dress design from European farm women's apparel.

PEAU de SOIE (pō′ də swä′) Heavyweight, fine ribbed, lustrous fabric. Often used for bridal garments.

PEBBLE FINISH Embossed finish on leather or vinyl that looks like tiny pebbles or rocks.

PEDAL PUSHERS *see* Pants

PEDS Small stocking footlet worn on foot with no outer appearance when covered by shoe.

PEIGNOR (pen′ wär) Women's decorative robe, usually designed to be worn with matching nightgown.

PENCIL SKIRT Very narrow, women's skirt, without flare.

PENCIL STRIPE Very narrow stripe woven in fabric.

PENDANT Ornament of jewelry, often placed on a chain and worn as a necklace. Also, dangling earrings.

PENNY LOAFER *see* Shoes

PEPLUM Small, full flare over skirt, covering hip area. Used in jackets, skirts, and dresses.

PERCALE Fabric of plain weave, combed cotton. Used in apparel and home furnishings.

PERMANENT PRESS A "finish" applied to fabrics through chemicals and heat treatment, to maintain a nonwrinkled look. Often used on cottons.

PETAL SLEEVES *see* Sleeves

PETER PAN COLLAR *see* Collars

PETITE SIZES Size range for women 5′4″ and under, with shorter bodice, sleeve, and skirt. Also size Small.

PETIT POINT (pet′ē point) Small needlepoint embroidery done on small canvas or mesh backing.

P

88

PETTICOAT Undergarment for woman or girl. Garment extends from waist to established hem, usually full or tiered, with lace, ruffles, or other adornment.

PICOT (pē′ kō) Decorative trim on edge of fabric, made of small loops. Made by hand or machine.

PICTURE *see* Hats

PIERROT (pye rō′) From French comedy character. Clownlike.

PIERROT COLLAR *see* Collars

PIGSKIN *see* Leathers

PIGTAIL Side or back braids of hair.

PILLBOX *see* Hats

PILLING Small hard surface balls of fabric, usually found in "wear" areas of garment, caused by use of staple yarns and/or loosely woven yarns.

PIMA COTTON Fiber of finer quality cotton with longer fibers.

PIN 1. Ornamental piece of jewelry with fastener on back to join pieces of cloth. Made of various metals, with or without gems or imitation stones. Often used at neckline on women's blouse, dress, or lapel. 2. Utilitarian piece of metal to hold fabrics together, either safety or straight pin.
Brooch Synonym for pin.
Cameo Facial silhouette carved from onyx or other layered gem, mounted in pin setting.
Clip Similar to pin but with spring clasp and snaps over edge of fabric.
Collar pin Fastened through eyelets in points of shirt collar.
Kilt pin Ornamental safety pin worn on kilt skirt.
Stick pin Straight ornamental pin, usually with design or jewel at top, and closure at bottom to hold into place.

PINAFORE Women's sleeveless garment, usually with dirndl skirt, bib top, and shoulder ruffle. Made into a dress or jumper. Wide use in childrenswear.

PINCHECK Fabric design of very small colored checks, woven or printed.

PINWALE Fabric of pile weave with narrow striped appearance, achieved through manufacturing process. Typically in corduroy.

PIPING Decorative edging made by sewing a fold of bias fabric usually over narrow cording, to the edge. Generally of contrasting color.

PIQUÉ (pē kā′) Fabric woven with ribbed and honeycomb design.

PLACKET Finished edge for a slit in the fabric of a garment. Typically found at the neckline or sleeve/cuff area.

PLAID Rectangular design woven or printed onto fabric and distinguished by multicolored yarns crossed at right angles. Includes madras and East Indian plaid that typically bleeds into fabric; argyle, a diamond design of various colors; glen, a large and small plaid-on-plaid design in similar, harmonious color; windowpane, a plaid of narrow cross stripes of color widely spaced to achieve window appearance; and tartan, plaids of distinctive patterns, identifying various Scottish clans through use of colored designs.

PLAIN WEAVE Fabric construction of interlaced yarns at right angles. Most used and least expensive construction.

PLAIT (plāt) Hairpiece added to hair, such as a braid.

PLASTIC Man-made materials from chemicals. Can be shaped or molded, low cost to manufacturer. Large usage in accessories.

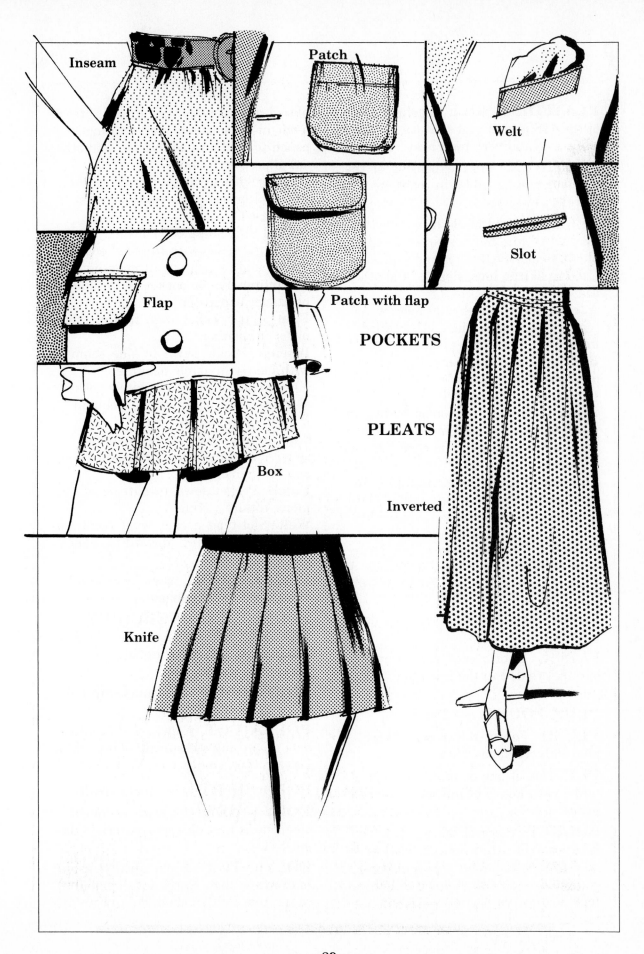

Inseam

Patch

Welt

Flap

Slot

Patch with flap

POCKETS

PLEATS

Box

Inverted

Knife

PLATFORM SOLE Fashion shoe of the 1960's and past centuries, with thick sole and very high heel.

PLATINUM Most expensive of the precious metals, silver in color. *see* Metals, Jewelry.

PLEAT A fold of cloth, stitched or unstitched into hard or soft pressed pleats to achieve design and fullness. Used in skirts, tops, sleeves, and other areas.

Accordian Pleat that is narrow at top, graduating to wider. Also called umbrella or sunburst pleat.

Box Double pleat, partially stitched or unstitched. Formed by two folds that meet in the center.

Crystal Narrow version of accordian pleat. Commonly used in bridalwear.

Engineered Pleat planned for a specific area of garment.

Fortuny Type of long, multiple, unsewn pleats that have the look of the original pleating process invented by Spanish designer, Mariano Fortuny.

Inverted Opposite side of box pleat with no folds visible from outer side.

Kick Small knife or other pleat at lower edge of skirt.

Knife Single fold of fabric used as a pleat.

PLISSÉ Fabric with a puckered surface created in the finishing process.

PLUS FOURS *see* Pants

PLUSH Fabric woven with warp pile. Velvety appearance.

PLY Use of one or more yarns to make yarn heavy or lighter for appropriate use.

POCKET Piece of fabric used for decorative or utilitarian purpose, to hold money and other objects. Placed on outside or inside of apparel and may or may not be visible. Origin placed in the sixteenth century, first as a slit in the garment into an inner pouch to hold a handkerchief and other small personal items.

Bellow/Safari/Cargo Patch pocket with center box pleat that expands when used.

Bound/Slot/Slash/Slit Pocket is inside of garment, with finished edges visible and forming a slit opening.

Envelope Patch pocket with side pleats for expansion.

Flap Inner pocket with flap of fabric to cover opening.

Inseam Pocket sewn to side seam with nearly invisible opening.

Kangaroo Very large patch pocket sewn in center of garment, frequently used to keep hands warm.

Key Small patch pocket usually sewn near waistband and used to hold keys or coins.

Patch Pocket sewn to outside of garment, totally visible.

Welt Slot-type pocket with rectangular fabric extending upward to cover opening.

POCKETBOOK Synonym and older word for handbag.

POCKET HANDKERCHIEF/SQUARE Small rectangle of fabric, usually silk, placed in upper jacket pocket for accent.

POINT LACE Lace made by needlepoint method.

POLKA DOT Fabric with colored dots of varying sizes printed onto cloth.

POLO COAT *see* Coats

POLO SHIRT *see* Shirts, Knit

POLYAMIDE Related chemical compounds that describe generic nylon. *see* Nylon.

POLYESTER A chemically made man-made fiber. Early development came from British chemists in the late

1930's. In 1946 du Pont purchased the rights to produce this fiber in the United States. By 1951, they manufactured the fiber into a yarn called Dacron®. Subsequently other companies named their polyesters.

As in all man-made fibers, it is first produced as a filament yarn and then may be cut into staple form. Polyester is very versatile and can be made to look like other yarns or fabrics, and has a great use in blends for wrinkle resistance. Other characteristics include lack of shrinkage, hydrophic (absorbs little moisture), and easy care.

Polyester fabrics are subject to static electricity and to absorbing oil stains. Polyester has good resistance to sunlight and a new development is fire retardant polyester sleepwear for infants. Another new development is a soil release, breathable polyester, under the trademark VISA®.

The newest development in polyester is termed "microfibers," a yarn that is much finer than the sheerest of sheer nylon stockings. Characteristics include its warmth, elasticity, and hand. Designers are producing jackets and suits to rainwear with microfibers.

POMPADOUR Hairstyle achieved by brushing hair high and smooth from forehead. Named for Madame Pompadour of France.

PONCHO Square or rectangular body cover, with slit or other head opening. Can be wool for warmth or vinyl for waterproof rain protection.

PONGEE Fabric with typical beige color and crisp hand, usually silk.

PONYTAIL Hairstyle achieved by pulling hair to center back of head and securing with elastic or other band. Hair is left falling down, as in a pony's tail.

POODLECLOTH Fabric knitted or woven with curled surface.

POODLE SKIRT Full, circle skirt from 1950's. With poodle dog design on surface.

POPLIN Fabric of firm weight and small rib.

POUCH *see* Handbags

PRÊT-À-PORTER (pre tȧ pôr tā′) French words for ready-to-wear.

PRINCESS STYLE Body-forming silhouette characterized by lengthwise panels and a flared skirt. Used in women's dresses and coats.

PRINT Designs printed onto fabric, produced by mechanical or hand method. Typically floral or geometric.

PRIVATE LABEL Merchandise that is manufactured for a specific retail store's specification and is labeled with the name of the store or a specific name chosen by the store.

PUFF Roundlike garment design produced by gathered fabric. Examples are puff sleeve and puff skirt. Also called a bubble skirt.

PULLON Pant or skirt without a zipper or other opening, with a stretch waistband, used in place of other openings.

PULLOVER Sweater without center front or other opening, pulled over the head and arms into place.

PUMPS *see* Shoes

PURITAN COLLAR *see* Collars

PURSE Synonym for handbag.

PVC Initials used for leatherlike plastic. Full name is polyvinylchloride. Used in making accessories and apparel. Inexpensive and easy care properties.

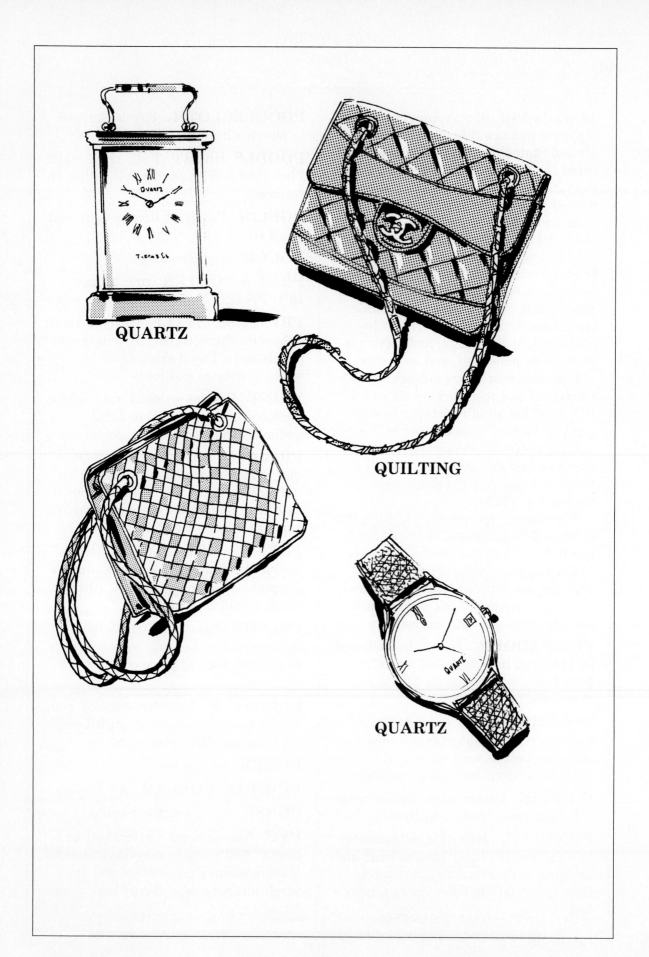

QUARTZ

QUILTING

QUARTZ

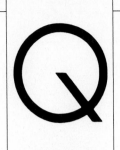

QUARTZ *see* Gems

QUARTZ WATCH One that is powered by vibrations of a quartz crystal which vibrates when charged by a special tiny battery. Extremely accurate timing.

QUEEN SIZE Sizing for larger women's pantyhose.

QUEUE (kyoo) *see* Hairstyles

QUILT Quilted fabric made into apparel. Quilted fabric has a face (outer or fashion) fabric, filling material such as polyester fiberfill or a natural material, such as down for insulation, and backing fabric. Layers are sewn together in selected areas to keep all the fabrics together. Often in a decorative design.

R

RAG BUSINESS/GAME
Slang for "apparel industry."

RAGLAN *see* Sleeve

RAINCOAT Waterproof or water resistant coat. Made waterproof if coated with plastic, plastic/vinyl, or rubber (slicker). An "all-weather" coat is an outer raincoat with a zip-out fleece or quilted lining for extra warmth. Regular raincoats are classic design, buttoned, made of poplin or other firm fabric, and given a water repellant finish. Trenchcoats were inspired by the military raincoat of World War I, usually double-breasted, with epaulets and a D-ring belt.

RAMIE Also called "China grass." Natural fiber obtained from the stalk of a plant in the nettle family. Stalks are processed by soaking in water or chemical means. Outer layer is stripped to obtain the fiber. Ramie has many linen characteristics, is a less expensive fiber, and is used in many blends with cotton. Current major use is in sweaters.

RASCHEL Machine which does a variety of fabric construction including knitted laces, power net, regular net, to heavy duty fabrics.

RATINE Similar to boucle. *see* Novelty Yarns.

RAWHIDE Untanned hide of animal.

RAW SILK *see* Silk

RAYON Known as "artificial silk," the first man-made fiber. Attributed to Count Hilaire de Chardonnet in France, 1891. Use of cotton linters or wood pulp, dissolved chemically and put through the spinnarette to obtain fiber. Officially named rayon (ray of sun) in 1924. Varieties include viscose rayon from purified cellulose (wood pulp). Is somewhat cottonlike, low in strength and resiliency, and high in absorbency. Can be dry cleaned, may be laundered. Used in blends, apparel, linings, and household items. Cuprammonium is no longer manufactured in the United States. High-wet Modulus rayon has greater stability when wet, more crisp hand, and used for apparel.

READY-TO-WEAR, R-T-W Apparel made in factories to standard size measurements. In the early 1800's, menswear was the first manufactured apparel. In the late 1800's, womenswear was made. Limited to nonfashion apparel. By the 1920's, designed, manufactured, and accepted as fashion apparel.

RECURRING FASHIONS Fashion of silhouettes that recycle into a current fashion look.

RECYCLED/REPROCESSED WOOL *see* Wool

REEFER *see* Coat

REMNANT Leftover fabric on bolt. Varying lengths, usually sold at a discount price.

REP Fabric with larger rib variation, of various fibers.

RESIDENT BUYING OFFICE Organization, housed in a major fashion market area, that covers the market, offers merchandising services, store planning, and computerization to a group of noncompeting retail stores that pay for this service.

RESIST PRINTING Coating areas of fabric to prevent absorption of dye. Materials of resist include starch, clay wax, and string. Batik is a wax resist process; tie and dye is to tightly

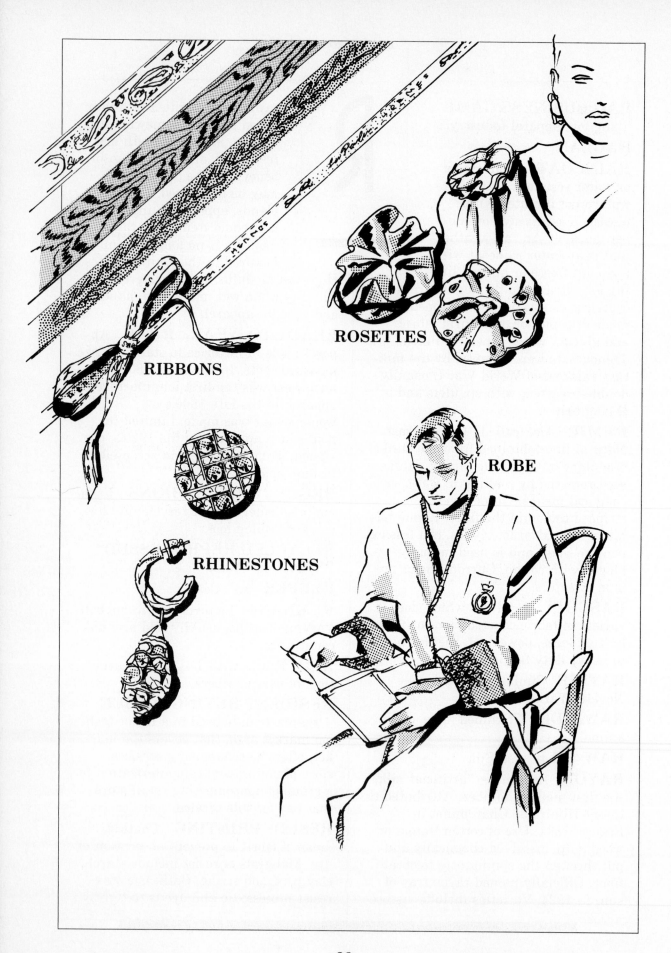

RIBBONS

ROSETTES

RHINESTONES

ROBE

tie areas to resist dye; and ikat is a method of warp resist dyeing. *see also* Ikat.

RETAIL Selling of items to consumers.

RETAILER Individual, store, or corporations that sell to consumers.

RETTING Process of decomposing outer layers of stalk of bast fiber, through the use of water or chemicals, to obtain inner fiber.

REUSED WOOL *see* Wool

RHINESTONE Colorless, artificial gem of paste or glass. Facets cut to sparkle like diamonds. Costume jewelry.

RIBBON Narrow strip of fine, decorated, ribbed fabric. Used as a trim, to hold hair in place, or as a sash.

RIB KNIT *see* Knit

RIDING HABIT *see* Equestrienne

RING Circular band, often decorated with gems, that encircles the finger (or toe). Fashion rings can be metal, metal and gems, small to very large, double or triple as in wedding rings, or solitaire, with a single stone.

RISE 1. Stage of fashion cycle after the Introduction of a new design, when it begins to be accepted by a small group of individuals, usually at a higher price level. 2. Measurement of pants, from crotch to waist.

ROBE Large, loose, unstructured garment. In nightwear, worn over nightgown or pajamas, and called a bathrobe. A wrap-style kimono is very popular for men and women. Also for women, the zip and button styles. Knee or long length, lightweight to heavy for warmth. May be short, worn in bed for top warmth or decor, called a bedjacket. *see also* Peignoir.

ROLLER PRINTING Use of engraved rollers, each a different color, through which fabric is passed and designs are applied. Most common, least expensive method of printing fabric.

ROSEPOINT *see* Lace

ROSETTE Roselike object, usually made of fabric to resemble a rose. Used to decorate garments or accessories.

ROVING Fibers in loose, untangled stage, just before spinning into yarn.

S Denotes size small, symbol "S" in women's and menswear, when sizing is not labeled in numbers. Is a more approximate sizing method.

SA Seventh Avenue, New York. The apparel, and accessory design and production center of the garment industry in the United States.

SABLE Russian animal of weasel family, noted for silky, dark blue-brown quality fur.

SADDLE SHOULDER Yoke-look in the shoulder or front of sweater, with raglan seam from underarm to yoke seam area.

SAFARI LOOK Adaptation of apparel worn by hunters on safaris in Africa, complete with wide-brimmed hat, cotton shirt, and pants with many pockets.

SAFFRON An orange dye color and cooking spice produced from the dried orange stigma of the crocus plant.

SALON SELLING Personal selling, bringing merchandise to an outer room to show customer. Usually elegant in decor. Examples: Designer's salon, fur salon.

SANDAL Shoe with sole, attached to foot with thongs, laces, or small straps. Sandals were first worn by ancient Egyptians, also Greeks and Romans. Most common sandal has a thong between first two toes of the foot. Huarache is a type of Mexican sandal. Sandals may be flat or high-heeled, may be attached at the ankle and foot (anklestrap). Made of leather, rubber, vinyl, plastics, metallics and various materials.

SAPPHIRE *see* Gems

SARI (sä′ rē) Fine, outer dresslike garment. One length is wrapped over waist to form skirt, other end is wrapped over head/shoulders. Worn by Indian/Pakistan women. Of Hindu origin.

SARONG Length of cloth wrapped around body at waist, hangs as a skirt. Of South Pacific origin.

SASH Length of fabric worn around waist as decor or to hold a wrapped garment together.

SATCHEL *see* Handbag

SATEEN Variation of satin weave with filling yarns as floats over warp yarn. Usually of fine cotton, not as lustrous as satin fabric.

SATIN 1. A weave, having intervals when warp yarns float over several filling yarns. Much of the beauty of satin weave is use of more loosely twisted yarns to reflect light and use of fibers that are more lustrous. 2. Lustrous fabric of satin weave, of silk, acetate, or other fiber. Satin fabric is more apt to snag, is less durable.

Types of satins: crepe back satin, lustrous face yarns, creped/twisted filling yarns, back of fabric is less lustrous with creped look, and face of fabric is lustrous; antique, made to look like aged satin; double face satin, use of two warps, one filling, lustrous on both sides of fabric; peau de soie, (pō′ də swä′) closely woven, less lustrous fabric; and slipper, strong fabric, often used for shoe uppers.

SCALLOP Curved, ornamental border on fabric or lace.

SCARF Square, rectangular, or triangular fabric worn at neck and/or over shoulders, usually for adornment, also for warmth or protection. Of silk, polyester, wool, cotton, and other fibers.

SCHIFFLI *see* Embroidery

SCOOP *see* Necklines

SCOTCH PLAID *see* Tartans

SCREEN PRINT/SILK SCREEN PRINTING Method of printing by hand or machine. A screen is used for each design. All areas of the screen design are blocked off except the area of the design which contains a certain color. A screen is prepared for each color and dye is rolled over the screen with the appropriate color. Screen was formerly a silk net, now of polyester or other material.

SEA ISLAND COTTON Quality, long staple cotton fiber.

SEAM Sewing two pieces of fabric together by hand or machine near their edges by fitting, joining, lapping, or other methods.

SEAM BINDING/TAPE Narrow, ribbonlike tape sewn over raw edge of fabric that has been turned up for hemming, to conceal raw edge of fabric.

SEAM FINISH Methods that seal raw edges of fabric in seams and prevent raveling. Overlock is a popular industry seam finish. Others are use of French seam, flat fell seam, zig zag, or turn to inside top stitch finish.

SEAMSTRESS Older term. *see* Dressmaker.

SECONDS *see* Irregulars

SEED HAIR FIBERS Fibers that grow from seeds that are formed in pods on certain plants. *see also* Cotton; Kapok.

SEERSUCKER Fabric with crinkled appearance. In manufacturing process, some warp yarns are held at tight tension, some at slack tension.

The slack areas puff up to create the permanent effect.

SELF COVERED Covering of the belt and/or buttons in matching fabric to garment.

SELVAGE/SELVEDGE (sel' vij) Edges of fabric woven so that it will not ravel.

SEMIPRECIOUS *see* Gems

SEPARATES Nonrelated items of casual clothing; pants, sweaters, tops, skirts, etc. When related by fabric and color are called "coordinates."

SEQUIN Small, shiny plastic disks, silver, black, or colored, with hole in middle and sewn to fabric for decorative, elegant effect. *see* Embellishment.

SERICIN Gummy substance extruded by silk worm when silk fiber is simultaneously extruded and hardens to hold it all together in the cocoon stage. Removed with a soap solution before or after fabric is woven. When a portion is left in fabric, it is called raw silk.

SERICULTURE The controlled production of silk through controlled growth and feeding of silk worms. Some are permitted to live and breed, and the remaining largest and heaviest worms are subjected to dry heat to kill the pupa. Silk fiber is obtained by soaking the cocoon and unwinding the filament in a process termed "reeling." Filament yarn from four or more cocoons forms a strand of silk yarn.

SET-IN *see* Sleeves

SEW To join one or more pieces of fabric, stitching by hand or machine.

SHANK 1. Part of sole of shoe under instep of feet. 2. Projection, either of thread or an attachment on back of button, leaving an extension for buttoning heavier fabric.

SHANTUNG (shan′ tuŋ′) Plain weave fabric with nubby, irregular filling yarn for texture effect.

SHAWL Square or oblong, decorative or utility, worn over head and shoulders. Small to very large; knit or woven.

SHAWL COLLAR *see* Collars

SHEARING To remove hair or fleece by cutting or clipping.

SHEATH *see* Dresses

SHEER Thin, fine, or transparent; a fabric industry term.

SHELL *see* Blouses

SHETLAND Quality wool from sheep of Shetland Islands. Of Scottish origin.

SHIRRING Gathering fabric into three or more parallel lines, for decorative effect.

SHIRT, CASUAL In recent years, the casual shirt of woven fabric was developed, and is usually worn without a tie. Many colorful styles, with short or long sleeves, colorful prints, Hawaiian prints, basic plaid/western, safari style, plain camp shirt, and worn either tucked in waist of pants or outside of pants. Worn by men and women. Body shirts developed for women, with long tails in both front and back that extend to, and snap at, the crotch.

SHIRT, DRESS Men's garment for upper part of body, having collar, sleeves, and opening. Evolved from the simple tunic, in medieval times. By the 1600's, had become very decorative, with lace at neck, large sleeves tied with ribbons, and of fine linen fabric. In the 1700's, continued to be of fine linen, ruffled front, and with small standing collar. The jabot was added to the front.

In the 1800's, men's shirts became plainer, though some had fancy front trims. The starched collar was introduced by Beau Brummell. By 1880, men's shirts altered in design and resemble the basic cut of today's shirts. Shirt variations include regular or French cuffs, pointed, spread or round collars, plain, colored, or striped fabrics, and worn with a tie.

SHIRT, FORMAL *see* Tuxedo

SHIRT, KNIT *see* Knitted Apparel

SHIRTWAIST First developed as a women's blouse in the 1890's with leg-of-mutton sleeves and high, banded collar. Gradually elongated to dress length and has been a popular garment for several decades. Now a dress of many fabrications, styled as an elongated, tailored shirt, worn belted or non-belted, and usually with a centered, buttoned closure.

SHOES Covering for the human foot. Shoes have been worn since earliest times. The simple Egyptian sandal and the Greek sandal with straps that crisscrossed around the foot, became elaborate by 400 B.C., some of leather covered with gold. Roman shoes covered the foot. In earliest medieval times, the shoe was of leather and laced together, followed by a man's shoe with excessively long and pointed toe, called the crackow. This pointed shoe was replaced with the broad-toe duck's bill. Since women's feet had been nearly invisible under long skirts, slippers had been worn.

A raised heel for women was introduced in the sixteenth century, some decorated with rosettes. Men of this time wore pumps that covered to the ankle. Footwear of the 1700's was highly decorated and continued the use of the heel. By the mid and late 1800's, men's shoe design was similar to to-

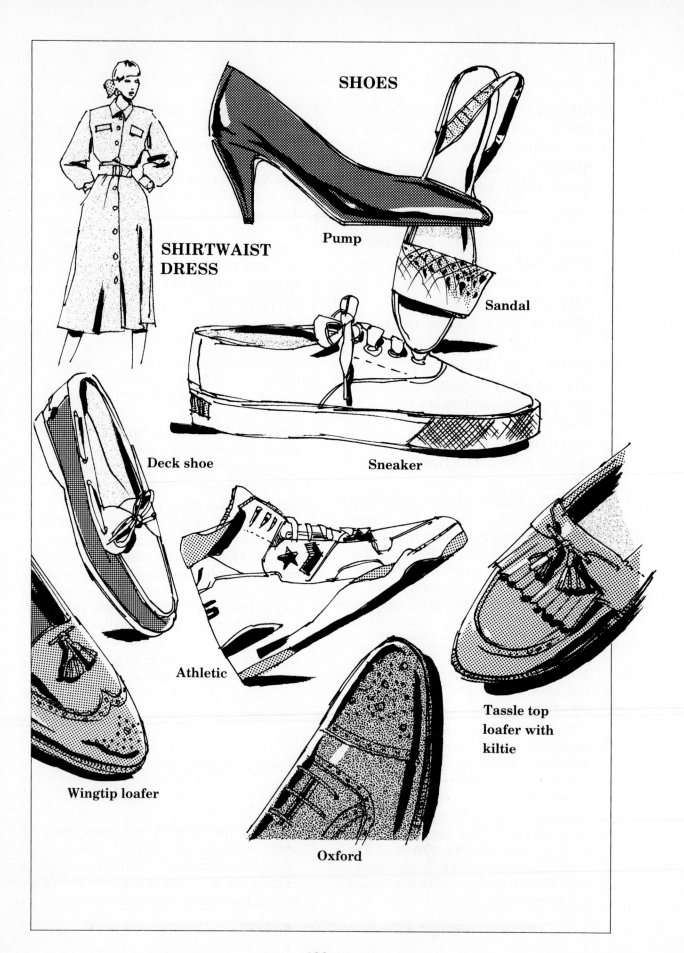

SHOES

SHIRTWAIST
DRESS

Pump

Sandal

Deck shoe

Sneaker

Athletic

Tassle top
loafer with
kiltie

Wingtip loafer

Oxford

day's oxford shoe. The high top of the 1900's women's shoes had many buttons and a pointed toe. Today's shoes vary widely in price, choice of materials, and design. Main categories of shoes:

Oxford Below the ankle, full shoe with center lacings. Some with decorated toe, wing tips, or with solid toe; saddle shoe, two-tone with dark color at center sides and back strip; and granny oxford, a higher, over the ankle oxford, copying the style of the 1900's.

Pumps Slip-on shoes for women, usually covering heel, sides and toes of foot. Many varieties, colors, fabrications, and designs, including the ballerina skimmer, a simple designed low heel pump; sling, a pump with a strap at top of heel and full heel opening; spectator, two color pump with a wing tip toe; evening pump, highly decorated in sequins, pearls, of special fabrics; espadrille, canvas summer shoe with mid high wedge heel of ropelike material; Mary Jane, low heel, black patent leather T-strap, little girl shoe; slide, shoe with high heels, full front but no heel covering; and tuxedo, men's formal patent leather shoe worn with a tuxedo.

Sandals Open shoes with a sole and straps, thongs, or other material to hold shoe to foot, with high or low heels. Many are low-heeled and colorful for summer season. Highly decorated women's sandals for evening occasions.

Slip-on More casual shoe for men and women without laces. Includes: loafer, modification of the mocassin with or without tassles; mocassin, look-a-like of soft Indian shoe; kiltie, a loafer with a fringed outer tongue and small decorative ties; dress oxfords, with decorative laces and side expandable gores for inserting the foot; and boat or deck shoe, loaferlike with non-skid soles and side lacing.

Sneaker Sports shoe with high or low tops, worn for athletic sports as well as casualwear. Most are white, some multicolored, may be of canvas, nylon, rubberized material, or combinations of materials. A variation is the water sock, with mesh uppers and rubberized sole, to be worn in water with rocks or other difficult walking surface.

SHOESTRING Fabric, leather, or other material strips to be used as lacing in shoes.

SHORT-RUN Production of a smaller amount of fabric than the norm.

SHORT-RUN FASHION Similar to a fad.

SHORTS Shortened pant with zipper, button opening, or elastic pull-on. Vary in length. Boxer shorts, with elastic waist; Bermuda, tailored appearance and long, to above the knee; athletic, lightweight, short, for sports; fuller shorts, resembling short, full skirts; and varying lengths from knee-length to very short athletic shorts. Hot pants were colorful women's shorts of the 1960's, worn instead of a mini skirt.

SHOULDER PAD Triangular or dolman style, rounded over the shoulder, pad with filler of foam or fiberfill, worn to extend the appearance of shoulders. Attached or velcro detachable and a totally detached one of foam, that is placed, and stays on the shoulder under the garment.

SIGNATURE Use of the designer's name imprinted on the merchandise; scarves, handbags, and others.

SILHOUETTE In fashion, the overall outline, or shape of a garment.

Three basic silhouettes form the basis for all clothing and are considered long-run fashions. These cycle over a period of years; the bell, with outer form rounded to waistline; the straight, hangs from the shoulders; and the bustle back silhouette. A-line and V-shape are modifications of the straight silhouette.

SILK Natural, filament fiber extruded from the cocoon after being constructed by the silkworm. Sericin is the gummy substance that holds the silk strands together in a cocoon form. Silk is reeled from cocoon into yarn for knitted and woven fabrics. Each cocoon contains 1 to 2000 feet of silk filament.

Silk is the strongest natural fiber, with some elasticity, good absorbency, and dyes beautifully. Sunlight and perspiration will deteriorate silk. Water spots are temporary and are removed when washed or drycleaned. When degummed, silk fabrics are lustrous and beautiful. When some gum (sericin) is left in, the fabric takes on a rough texture without luster termed raw silk and is used for suiting. Spun silk noil is fabric made of end pieces, with a dull texture and soft hand. Tussah is silk from a wild species, is a coarser fabric, and tan-colored. Occasionally, two silkworms will spin a cocoon together, producing a double strand of yarn called doupion silk. Sandwashed silk is a manufacturing process that slightly naps and dulls the silk. *see also* Sericulture.

SILVER *see* Metals, Precious

SINGLE-BREASTED Suit jacket or coat with center closure and a single line of button(s).

SINGLE KNIT *see* Knits, Jersey

SIZING 1. Starch, gelatin, or other material added to fabric for temporary body, which disappears after washing. Resin, when applied to fabric, produces a durable, firm finish. 2. Industry measurements as a guide for apparel sizes.

SKIRT Part of a garment that hangs from waist down or a separate garment that hangs from waist down. Worn by men and women in varying lengths from the earliest days. Cretan women wore a full-length bell skirt, while Egyptian men wore a short, often pleated skirt. Skirts worn by women during the centuries were usually a simple wrap style. In the 1700's, skirts were fuller and gathered into a waistband. The shirtwaist blouse of the 1890's was a very popular style and worn with a bell skirt. Dressier skirts were introduced as well as skirts with jackets—suits. Current skirt styles include:

A-line Skirt with flare, wider at hem than at hip.

Asymmetric Any off-center major design line in skirt.

Bell Skirt with some gathers at waist and full flare near hem.

Bouffant Fully gathered skirt.

Circle Full or half-circle skirt.

Culotte *see* Pants

Dirndl Skirt gathered at waist into waistband.

Draped Skirt of soft fabric that has been pulled into a side or front drape.

Gored Skirt made of lengthwise panels called gores. Minimum of four to many gores.

Hoop Large full skirt held out at hem with hoops or hooped slip. Current use in bridalwear.

Kilt Scottish tartan, wrap, fully pleated skirt with side fringe. Usually fastened with large ornamental safety pin. Worn by Scottish men for special events. Also made for women and children. Tartan used denotes the clan of the wearer.

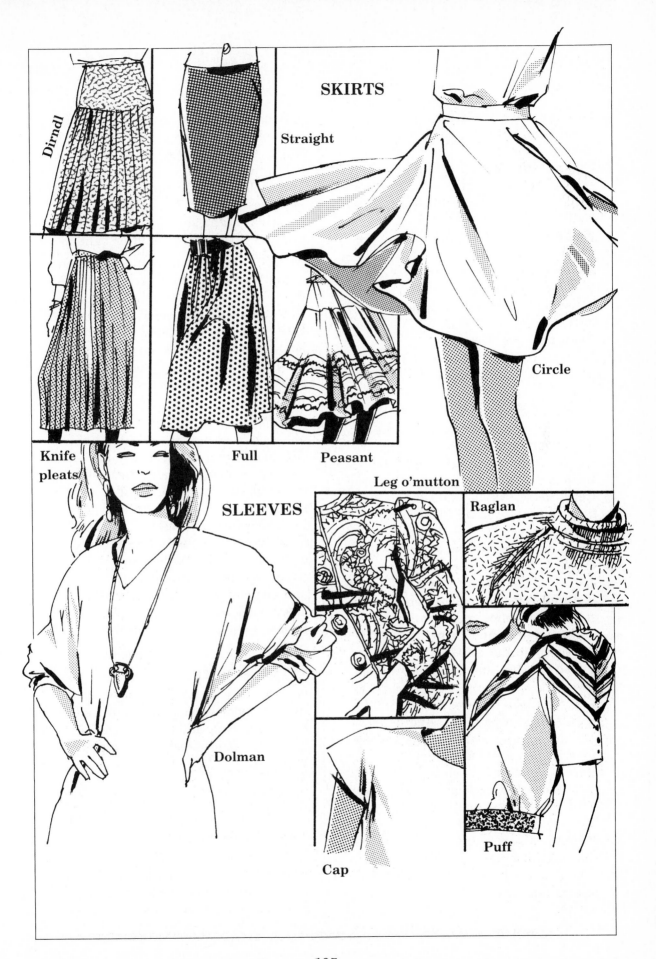

Dirndl

Straight

SKIRTS

Circle

Knife pleats

Full

Peasant

Leg o'mutton

SLEEVES

Raglan

Dolman

Cap

Puff

105

Peasant, prairie Fully gathered skirt, often with an additional gathered tier near hem.

Pencil, slim/straight Straight line skirt, fitting the waist and hip. Often with a slit or lower pleat so wearer can walk with comfort.

Pleated Any skirt with pleats. *see* Pleats.

Sarong Side draped skirt, usually of bright floral design.

Skort A skirt-pant variation. *see* Culottes.

Trumpet *see* Dresses

Wrap Length of fabric, wrapped around body, overlapped and secured at waist.

SLEEVES Part of garment that covers all or part of the arm. Can be utilitarian or decorative, of many lengths from cap to full length of arm. Includes:

Bell Sleeve which fits armhole and flares out at wrist, in bell-like appearance.

Cap Small extension of garment bodice to form slight covering for upper arm.

Dolman/Batwing All-in-one full sleeve and bodice, with center of arm seam and deep underarm, sometimes extending to the waist.

Fitted Sleeve that is shaped in the form of the arm.

Leg-o'mutton Sleeve of the 1900's with exaggerated fullness gathered at top and set into garment, from elbow to wrist becomes fitted in style.

Petal Short, set in sleeve with curved overlapped fabric in petal form.

Puff Full sleeve, gathered and set into armhole.

Raglan Sleeve designed with seams that extend from underarm to neckline in slanted style. Curved dart or seam shapes sleeve to shoulder of wearer.

Set-in Any sleeve which is sewn to armhole of garment.

Shirt Basic tailored set-in sleeve, with minimum fullness at shoulder, lower edge is fuller and gathered, and is stitched to cuff. The bishop is a variation of the shirt sleeve with more fullness gathered into cuff or band.

SLIP Lingerie worn under women's or girl's outer garment. *see also* Camisole.

Bra Slip with attached bra top.

Full Slip covering body from chest to hem, with thin straps over shoulders.

Half Slip from waist to hem, varying lengths, usually elastic band at waistline.

SLIPPERS Light, low shoes, usually worn indoors, of washable lightweight summer fabric, fleece for winter warmth or leather and/or fleece-lined for additional warmth. Scuff is a soft slipper covering toes, with or without heel covering. Soft leather is a man's loafer variation. Soft mocassins are also used as slippers by men. Quilted, bootlike slippers are worn by women and girls for warmth. Slipper socks are anklet socks with a thin, soft suedelike sole.

SLIT An opening in clothing.

SLOPER/BLOCK Tag board basic pattern made to body measurements. Includes bodice back and front, skirt back and front, and sleeve. Used as basis for pattern design development.

SMALL *see* S

SMOCK *see* Dresses

SMOCKING Type of needlework, gathering small bits of fabrics into decorative, colorful designs.

SNAKESKIN The thin skin of a reptile. Needs a backing for stability, used for accessories, such as belts, handbags, and shoes. Very distinctive markings; fragile.

SOCKS Knitted foot and/or leg covering.

Ankle/bobby Short sock, from foot coverlet to sock covering ankle. Usually of terry, may be plain or thin knit with lace edgings for little girls. Many brightly colored, patterned socks are also available.

Athletic/Crew/Tube Heavier terry sock, usually white, extends to calf. Some with colorful leg stripes. Recreational sport use, also.

Dress Men's lightweight sock worn with tailored suit, usually dark colored. Of many fibers including wool, nylon, and blends.

Knee-hi Sock with attached leg to just below kneecap.

SOFT GOODS/LINES Fashion industry term for apparel, accessories, and domestics (kitchen/bath/bedroom fabrics). *see also* Hard goods/lines.

SOLUTION DYED When color is added to the liquid form of the man-made fiber solution before extrusion. Extremely color fast, but more limited range of colors.

SOUTACHE *see* Braid

SPANDEX Man-made elastomeric fiber with extensive stretch and recovery. Stronger and more lasting than rubber. Generally resistant to mild chlorine and not affected by sea water. Used as a core yarn, covered with nylon, polyester, cotton or other, depending on ultimate use. Used in swimwear, bras, control pantyhose, recreational sports clothing, and others.

SPECIALTY STORE Store with a defined target customer which carries limited merchandise for that customer. Can be both large or small.

Usually more customized and personal services.

SPENCER *see* Jackets

SPINNERETTE Sievelike device that man-made liquid is forced through in the process of fiber making.

SPINNING Taking strands of fibers and twisting them together to produce yarn or thread.

SPLIT Horizontal separation of leather into layers. Splits, the inner layers, are of lesser quality than the top or outer layer.

SPORTSWEAR Clothes for comfortable, casual wear. Not recreational.

STAPLE Fibers of short lengths.

STIRRUP *see* Pants

STOLE Decorative scarflike accessory, of fabric or fur, worn over shoulders.

STRAW Stalks from grain, made into hats, totes, and other items.

STRETCH Use of one of several methods to obtain stretch and recovery in garments. 1. Core fiber of spandex. 2. Bicomponent, or two formula fibers. 3. Chemically crimped fibers.

STRIPES Horizontal or vertical, thin to wide, bands of colors. Pinstripe is a very narrow band of color.

STYLE 1. Distinctive appearance of a garment due to design, fabrication, etc. Some styles are so specific that they are named for a period in history, such as Greek or Victorian. 2. A number assigned to a specific item of merchandise.

SUEDE CLOTH Fabric that has had fiber ends brushed up into a low pile on the surface (not a pile fabric).

SUIT Jacket, trousers, or skirt that match in color and fabric. Optional item is the addition of a vest. Men's suits evolved in the 1830's with the general acceptance of long stirrup pants by men, with jacket cut in straight lines, and having back tails. Suit jackets gradually changed to current styles. Pants are straight legged, without stirrups. Women's suits of various styles were worn in the early 1900's. Chanel introduced the dressmaker suit in the 1920's. Current suits include:

Formal Tuxedo, men's formalwear. Black, grey, or to fashion colors of the period. Jacket is single- or double-breasted, with shawl or notched collar often of satin, tailored pant, and optional vest and fabric cummerbund. Jacket may be short, suit length, or with long back tails.

Tailored Classic suits for men and women, single- or double-breasted, notched or peaked lapel, with or without back vents. Men's single-breasted suits often have a matching vest. Women's suits may have a matching skirt or tailored pant. Generally of wool or wool blend. Considered a classic business look.

SUITING Durable fabrics used for men's and women's suits, usually firmly woven wool or wool blend.

SUMPTUARY LAWS Laws that regulate apparel and accessories as to size, height, elegance, or color. May be by religious organizations, laws of kings or queens, or by public ordinances.

SUNBURST *see* Pleat, Accordian

SUNGLASSES Eyeglasses with tinted or polarized lens to protect from sun. For frame styles, *see* Glasses.

SURPLICE *see* Dresses

SUSPENDERS/BRACES Detachable straps worn over shoulders, buttoned to front and back of pant to hold in place. Can be very decorative.

SWEATBAND 1. Exterior band of absorbent fabric, usually terry, worn over forehead and around head to absorb sweat when in a recreational sports event. 2. Inner band of man's hat to protect hat from sweat, of leather or fabric.

SWEATERS Outerwear, knitted garment of wool, mohair, cashmere, cotton, blends, or man-made wool-like fibers, worn on upper part of body, usually for additional warmth. Handmade or machinemade. Sweaters became fashionable when worn by male golfers in the 1920's with "plus fours." Women's elegant evening sweaters were designed by Schiaparelli in the 1930's.

Current sweaters are designed in two main styles: Pull over/on—Sweater with opening for head and pulled on over head. May have crew, turtle, cowl, or V neck. Cardigan—A sweater with button or zip front opening. Also called a coat sweater, with or without a collar.

Styles of sweaters include:

Embellished Part or all is decorated with beading, sequins, appliqué, other.

Fair Isle Round, patterned design at neck/chest area. Originally hand knit by women of Fair Isles (Scotland). Now hand or machine made and patterned area is attached to sweater blocks.

Fisherman's Knit/Aran Isle Large cable stitch identification. Originally hand knit by women of Aran Isles. Of Irish origin.

Golf Low, V neck, buttoned cardigan, style favored by golfers.

Jacquard Any patterned sweater made with jacquard attachment. Floral, geometrics, and others.

Shetland Originally fine wool from Shetland Isles (Scotland). Now synonymous with fine quality pull overs.

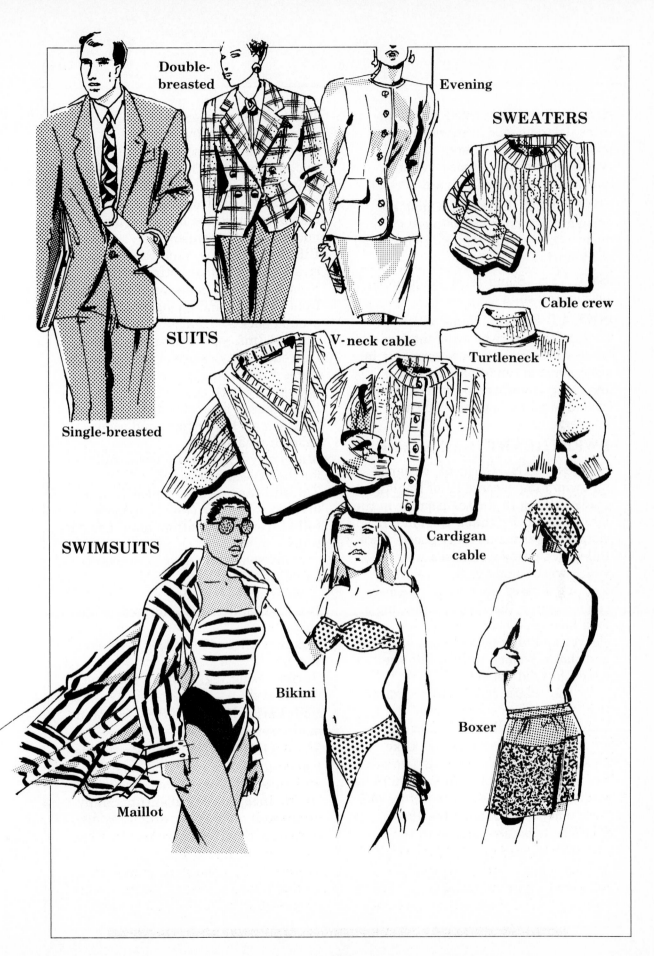

Double-breasted

Evening

SWEATERS

Cable crew

SUITS

V-neck cable

Turtleneck

Single-breasted

Cardigan cable

SWIMSUITS

Bikini

Boxer

Maillot

Ski Sweaters patterned from Fair Isles, Islandic, and other northern areas. Favored by skiers.

Vest Sleeveless, V neck sweater, pull over, or cardigan styles.

SWEATER DRESS One-piece elongated sweater or two-piece garment with sweater top and coordinated knit skirt.

SWEATS Slang term for jogging, or running suits.

SWEAT SHOP Name given to contractors (one who owns the business) whose workers sew garments in poor working conditions, with poor pay, long hours, and poor ventilation. Thus the name "sweaters" for the workers.

SWEETHEART *see* Necklines

SWIMSUITS Garment designed for swimming. George IV of England made bathing in the sea popular in the late 1700's at Brighton, England. In shapeless garments, court guests were rolled in chairs into the sea water, which was thought to be curative. Bathing dresses were worn by American women in the 1900's, consisting of long bloomers, belted dress with sleeves and high necks, black stockings and shoes. Women walked into the water, but did not swim.

By the 1920's, styles had been drastically altered to show more of the body, with thigh-length shorts and short skirt and sleeveless tanklike tops. Men had worn long leg, two-piece bathing suits, replaced in the 1920's by thigh-length trunks and tank tops. All were made of wool until the 1940's. Men's suits became topless in the 1930's. The two-piece suit emerged for women in the 1940's, followed by the bikini of the 1960's, a style of minimal top and bottoms. This emerged into a string bottom by the 1980's. Current styles are made from nylon/spandex blends, some cotton or cotton blends and include for women:

Bikini Two-piece suit. Bandeau or strap tops. Minimal bottoms with French cut legs. Some suits with small front covering and string attachment around back and waist.

Maillot (mä yō′) One-piece suit. Current leg styles are classic cut to extreme French (high) cut at sides. Styles vary with cut outs, minimal tops, blouson tops, strapless, bandeau tops, straps, halter tops, and some short draped skirts.

Maternity Suits with extra fullness for the expectant mother.

Tankini Sports suit copied from skin diver look. One-or two-piece, more fully covered top, bottom often has partially covered legs.

Many swimsuits also have coordinated cover ups.

Mens styles include:

Bikini Small trunks, formed to the body.

Boxer Pull on full boxer style shorts.

Surfer Long leg, colorful cotton trunks style.

SYNTHETIC FIBERS *see* Manmade, Petroleum base

SYNTHETIC GEMS Man-made. Identical in chemistry and crystal structure to natural gems. Begun in 1880's. Inexpensive substitute. Many are so well made, they cannot be discerned by the average consumer's eye.

TAFFETA Plain weave fabric, rib variation, made of filament yarn from acetate or silk, with slight sheen and slight rustle sound. Firm fabric.

TAILOR 1. Individual who makes garments such as suits and coats. 2. One who alters garments.

TAILORED CLOTHING Structured or semi-structured suits, coats, or overcoats. Both machine and some hand tailoring is used.

TALL Size designation of clothing for men over six feet tall.

TANK Knit, sleeveless, scoop neckline variation of T-shirt.

TANNING Treatment to animal skins to turn them into long lasting leather. Tannic acid was first used, and is found in oak bark. It still produces the finest, firmest leather. Chrome tanning is the quickest, least expensive method now in use.

TAPERED Gradually decrease in width; for example, in leg of pant.

TARTAN Name of any of numerous, distinctively colored plaid fabrics, worn by members of a Scottish clan. Better known tartans are the Black Watch, Stewart, and many more.

TASSEL Hanging ornament consisting of shorter lengths of threads, bound by a thread near one end. Used for embellishment.

TATTERSAL Fabric woven with dark lines forming checks on a lighter colored fabric.

TAUPE (tōp) Brownish, grey color.

TEDDY Decorative lingerie with an all-in-one camisolelike top and tap panty.

TENT *see* Dresses

TERRY CLOTH 1. Pile weave, looped fabric with two sets of warps and one filling. As filling is tightened, the warp loops into place. May be on one or both sides of fabric. 2. Pile knit looped fabric using two sets of yarns fed into knitting machine. One set loops up. Not as durable as woven terry but more flexible and comfortable.

TEXTILES 1. Cloth or fabric. 2. Fiber or yarn used to make cloth. (Textile Fiber Products Identification Act) (TFPIA), 1960 legislation requiring each textile product to have an attached label with the generic name of the fiber used by the percentage of weight. Fibers less than five percent are listed as "other." Amended in 1984 to require listing of country of origin.

THERMAL Garments or accessories worn for additional warmth; for example, underwear, socks.

THREAD Strands of fiber or filament of natural or man-made fiber used in garment construction.

TIARA (tē ar′ ə) Ornamental, crownlike headpiece. Often jeweled. Also used as bridal headwear with veil.

TIE 1. Long, colorful bias strip of fabric, wider at one end, of silk, polyester or blends, worn under shirt collar, hanging down in center front. Tied in knot at neck. Long ties use one of the following tieing methods:
Four-in-hand knot Wider end of tie crosses over narrow end two times and passes through loop, is drawn up to collar to tighten.
Half-Windsor knot Wider end of tie crosses over narrow and is brought up

111

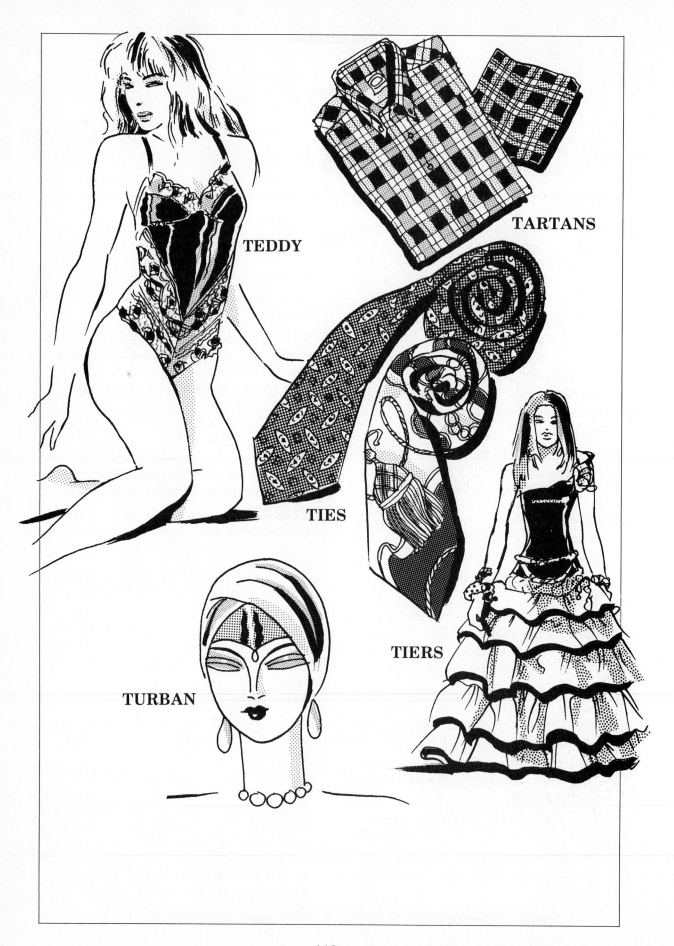

TEDDY

TARTANS

TIES

TIERS

TURBAN

112

and through loop, crosses again and passes through loop, drawn up to tighten.

Windsor Knot The widest variety. Wider end of tie crosses over front and through loop, then down, around narrow end, up and across front, through loop to tighten.

A short tie is called a Bow. Colorful short tie worn at neck under shirt collar, tied in bow at center front. Also clip-on style. Formal bow ties are black, white, colored, or metallic.

TIE CLASP Decorative, double metal bar used to hold tie to shirt front.

TIE PIN/TACK Small decorative pin with pointed center to go through tie and shirt and secure at back. Used to hold tie to shirt.

TIERS Gathered layers of ruffles to decorate bouffant skirts. Any type of layers of fabric on skirt to enhance design.

TIGHTS Snug fitting, knitted, all-in-one panty, leg, and foot cover. Used by dancers, for aerobics and other exercising, and some high wire circus performers. Usually opaque, often colorful, made of nylon/spandex blend.

TOGGLE *see* Closure

TOILE (twäl) Sheer fabric, used in fashion designing as a muslin sample design. Of French origin.

TONGUE Small part of shoe, used under lacings.

TOP Any casual type garment worn over top of body; for example, T-shirt, shirt, halter.

TOPAZ *see* Gems

TOPCOAT *see* Coat

TOP GRAIN Outer layer of animal hide or skin with distinctive hair markings. Considered the finest quality.

TOP HAT Formal hat with high, flat crown and narrow brim. Worn with tuxedo for formal occasions.

TOP STITCH Machine (sometimes hand) stitch on outside of garment, often for more interesting finished look.

TORSO Trunk of human body from neck to leg. Mannequins may also be in torso form rather than complete figure.

TORTOISE SHELL Mottled color look copied from sea turtle, used in accessory items such as eye glass frames, combs, and more.

TOTE *see* Handbag

TOUPEE (too pā') Men's hairpiece or partial wig, worn to cover bald spot on head.

TOW (tō) Weak fibers that have been straightened, with the shorter ones removed, and ready for spinning into yarn.

TRADE MAGAZINES/PUBLICATIONS Trade publications of the fashion industry include *Women's Wear Daily, Daily News Record, California Apparel News, W,* and other more specific to items; for example, *Footwear, Accessories,* etc. *see* Magazines, Fashion.

TRADEMARK Name or symbol identifying a product, officially registered and restricted, legally, to owner or manufacturer. For example, Dacron® is a specific polyester made by the du Pont Co.

TRAIN Long fabric, part of garment that follows along and trails behind wearer. Used in bridal wear and some formal wear.

TRANSLUCENT Partially transmitting light, to give perception of shape.

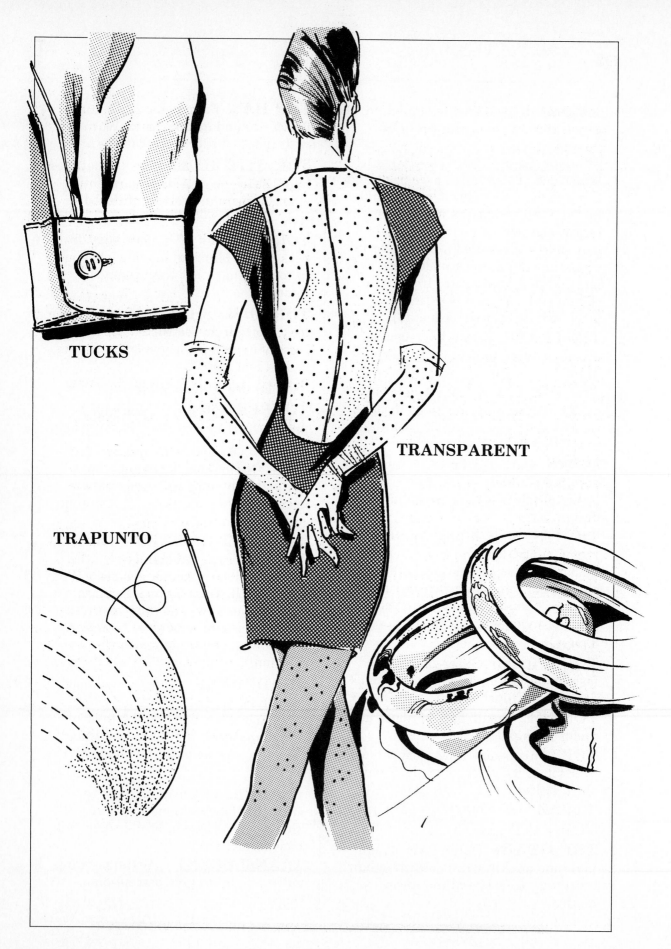

TUCKS

TRANSPARENT

TRAPUNTO

TRANSPARENT Capable of being totally see-through and sheer.

TRAPUNTO Hand or machine quilting, generally in rows, for a design effect.

TRENCHCOAT *see* Coats

TREND *see* Fashion

TRIACETATE Modified cellulose fiber, less absorbent than acetate, good wrinkle recovery and dimensional stability. Can be heat set into permanent pleats or other shapes. Can be washed or drycleaned. Used for apparel.

TRICOT (trē kō) Warp knitted fabric. Machine knit flat. Used extensively in lingerie, bonded backing to fabrics, and as shoe linings.

TROUSERS *see* Pants, Tailored

TRUMPET *see* Dresses

TRUNKS Loose leg, drawstring waist shorts. Worn extensively by men, boys, and some women. Originally worn by boxers.

TRUNK SHOW Designer, manufacturer, or designer's representative takes the newest sample line to a store to show customers and take orders. Test newest styles and colors for acceptability.

T-SHIRT *see* Knit, Apparel

TUCKS To make one or more small folds in fabric.

TULIP *see* Dresses

TULLE (tool) Very fine, sheer net. Used in bridalwear and ballet dancer's skirts.

TUNIC *see* Dresses

TURBAN Fabric wound around head. Of Muslim origin. Hat made in this design, fully covering head.

TURTLENECK *see* Necklines

TUSSAH *see* Silk

TUXEDO *see* Suits, Formal

TWEED Rough surface woolen, with several colors to obtain patterns, checks, or plaids. Used for suitings. Can also be a cotton tweed. Tweeds include:

Cheviot Warp and filling the same color.

Donegal Plain weave with colored slubs woven in.

Harris Imported, high quality Scottish wool from Harris Island.

Irish White warp, filling is darker color.

Scottish Homespun look.

TWENTIES LOOK *see* Flapper

TWILL WEAVE/FABRICS Strong, durable, compact weave. Fabric is identified by diagonal line on fabric. Warp face twill includes denim and gabardine. Herringbone twill reverses itself to form a broken diagonal line that appears as a VVV for decorative effect.

TWO-WAY STRETCH Knitted fabric with both horizontal and vertical stretch. Used extensively in swimwear.

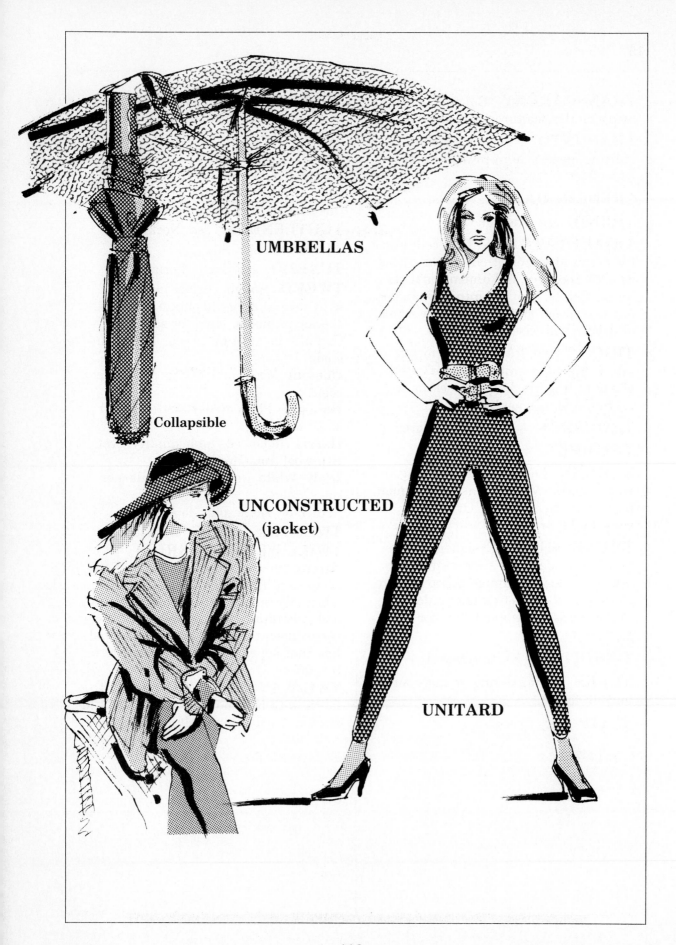

UMBRELLAS

Collapsible

UNCONSTRUCTED
(jacket)

UNITARD

U

ULTRASUEDE® Trade-mark of suedelike fabric, non-woven (felted) construction, of polyester and polyurethane. Used for jackets, dresses, and trims.

UMBRELLA Accessory item for protection from rain, consisting of collapsible can-opy of nylon mounted on a central rod with ribs to hold it in shape and decorative or functional handle. Types include fold-up and rigid construction. The fold-up styles are nine inches, regular and extra large. The rigid styles are regular and extra large. Umbrellas are black, colored, and multicolored. They are becoming a fashion item when purchased to match one's outerwear apparel.

UNDERSHIRT 1. Men's knitted cotton or cotton blend shirt, to be worn under outer clothing, with crew, V-, or U-neck, with or without short sleeves. 2. Infants knit-ted shirt, worn under clothing.

UNDERWEAR Overall term for clothing worn close to body and under outer garments.

UNITARD All-in-one bodysuit of stretch fabric covering torso and legs.

UNSTRUCTURED Casual, sports jackets with loose fit, little or no lin-ing, and no hand tailoring.

UPPER Part of shoe that fits over foot and is attached to sole.

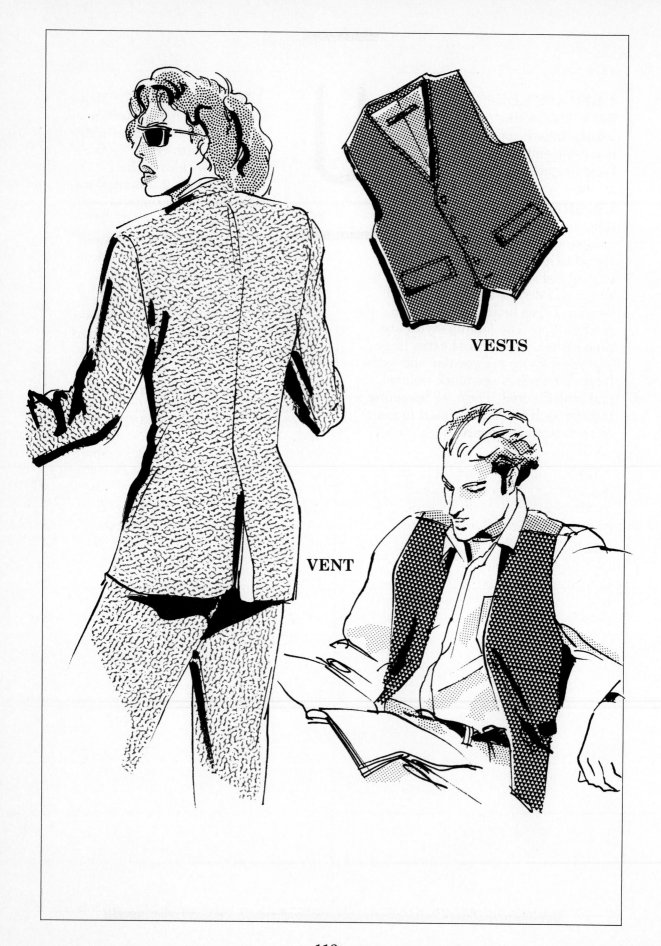

VESTS

VENT

118

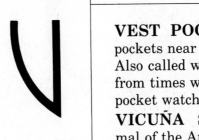

VAMP Part of shoe or boot covering the instep.

VEIL Net or lace used as trim on hat, part of bridal headwear, or placed on head as decorative accessory.

VELOUR Pile knit or woven fabric, using terry construction, then cut evenly for a soft velvety surface.

VELVET Woven pile fabric of silk or man-made fiber, cotton or rayon back, with short, soft thick luxurious surface. Crushed velvet has as special "ironed" appearance.

VELVETEEN Pile fabric with extra set of filling yarn, uniformly cut, commonly made of cotton.

VENDOR Resource. Supplier of merchandise.

VENT Vertical, faced slit, typically in men's suit jackets and coats, going from the hem, upward. Typically one or two in men's jackets.

VEST Short, form fitting sleeveless top. May be woven with button front to coordinate with single-breasted suit, may also be decorative and colorful. Also knitted with button front or pull over style.

VEST POCKET Welt pockets near waist of vest. Also called watch pocket, from times when men carried pocket watches.

VICUÑA Small, wild animal of the Andes Mountains. Hair fiber is used for apparel. Animal must be killed to obtain hair. Expensive and softest of fibers.

VINTAGE In fashion, the use of old, outmoded, classic apparel.

VINYL Plastic with leatherlike appearance. Used in footwear, handbags, wallets, and more. Also called "faux leather."

VISCOSE RAYON *see* Rayon

VISOR 1. Semicircular projection on cap to protect from sun. 2. Semicircular accessory item of plastic or material worn on forehead to protect from sun.

VISUAL MERCHANDISING Use of mannequins, torsos, props, cases, and walls to display merchandise in store or in outer windows of store.

VIOLE (voil) Sheer, soft, crisp finish, drapable fabric, made of cotton; man-made or blends.

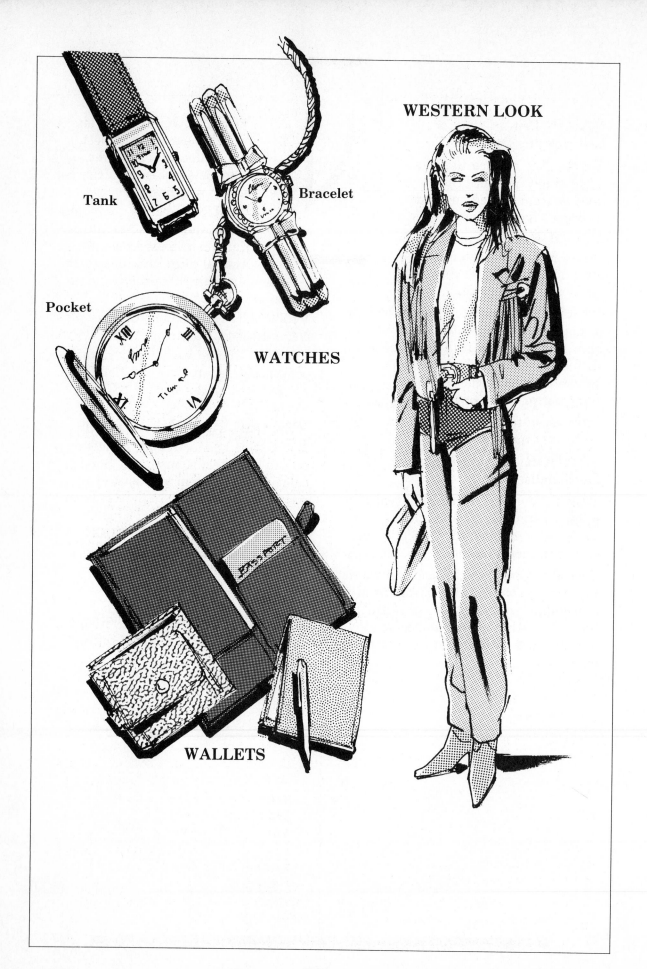

Tank

Bracelet

Pocket

WATCHES

WALLETS

WESTERN LOOK

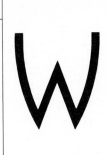

WAIST Mid or narrowest area of human body.

WAISTBAND Garment band encircling waist, seamed to a skirt or pant.

WAISTLINE Horizontal seam connecting bodice (top) and skirt. Natural waistline would be at the regular waist. Empire waistline is a high waist with seam below bust. Dropped waistline is lower than normal waist, seamed at hip area.

WALE 1. In corduroy, evenly spaced characteristic vertical strips, from narrow to wide, for decorative effect. 2. In knits, rows of stitches that run in columns in lengthwise direction.

WALLET Small accessory item used by men and women to carry money, drivers license, identification, credit cards, and more. Men's styles include: chest style, carried in inner top pocket of jacket. Double and triple fold, carried in hip pocket. Women's style may be much wider, usually containing an area for a check book and attached coin purse. Most wallets are made of leather or lesser priced vinyl, designer logo styles, fabric, nylon with velcro closing, and carried in a handbag.

WARDROBE All articles of clothing belonging to an individual.

WARP Lengthwise yarns used in weaving. Vertical direction in flat knitting.

WARP PRINT Unusual printing process with design printed onto warp yarns using roller printing process, then filling yarns are woven in. Effect is soft, shimmering patterns.

WATCH Watches have been in use for over 500 years. Current watches include two main types: analog, with numbers or stick figures, hour, and minute hand, and digital (since the early 1970's) with liquid crystal display (LCD) to show current time. Older watches used a windup method to keep them going. Current watches now use a quartz crystal with a vibrating bar charged by a special, tiny battery.

Cases used to hold watches are inexpensive, colored or black plastic, stainless steel, aluminum, or plated brass, gold or platinum, and may have precious stones. Watchband may be plastic, leather, or metal and is worn firmly at the wrist. Other styles include bracelet watches, pendant watches on neck chains, ring watches, pocket watches, and many trendy, unusual watches for all ages. Watch faces are round, oval, rectangular, and square.

WATERPROOF Water or moisture cannot penetrate. Use of plastic for garments or plastic coated fabrics.

WATER RESISTANT/REPELLENT Resists, but is not impervious to water. May have a finish to repel or shed water.

WEAVE Construction of fabric by interlacing yarns at right angles. Warp yarns are lengthwise, filling yarns are horizontal. Woven fabric is more stable, has little stretch, and may drape, depending upon fiber and yarn weight. Woven on complex mechanical looms. Can also be woven on hand looms.

Types of weaves:

Plain The interlacing of one yarn over another. Basket variation, interlacing two yarns over two or more combinations. Rib variation, using larger yarns in one direction for rib effect.

Satin weave The interlacing of yarns with warp floats over filling during construction. Identified by lustrous appearance, by reflecting light and sateen variation. More fragile.

Twill weave The interlacing of yarns in diagonal lines. Identified by diagonal line on surface, and herringbone variation. More tightly woven and strong construction.

A jacquard attachment is used to weave a pattern into the fabric. Pile weave is the use of additional warp or filling yarn so that yarn stands up or curls. Specialized machines produce decorative fabrics. *see also* Plain; Twill; Satin; and Jacquard.

WEDGE *see* Shoes

WEFT Filling or horizontal yarn in fabrics.

WESTERN LOOK Complete look with ten-gallon hat, plaid shirt, fringe vest, jeans, decorative belt, and boots. Many variations.

WET LOOK Garments with a watery or shiny look.

WICKING Moisture is not absorbed into the fiber (fabric or garment), but body moisture can escape and evaporate.

WIG Complete headpiece to cover head, of human hair or man-made fiber (modacrylic and others). Human hair is most costly.

WINDSOR *see* Ties

WING *see* Collars

WING TIP *see* Shoes

WOAD (wōd) Plant leaves formerly used to obtain blue dye.

WOMENS Size range for larger women, over 5'4", usually ranging from size 38 to 52.

WOOL Natural protein fiber obtained from sheep by shearing. Of various breeds and qualities, the Merino being the finest. Fleece (hair) sheared from eight month old sheep is called "lamb's wool" and is softer and finer. Wool removed from slaughtered animal is termed "pulled" wool, and is of lesser quality.

Characteristics of wool include: elasticity (has natural crimp), light in relation to weight, traps air to provide warmth, takes dye well, water repellent, but absorbent, and generally considered fire repellent. Has a tendency to felt and shrink, susceptible to moths, will deteriorate in sunlight, and is expensive depending upon quality. Some individuals are allergic to wool. Used for many types of outerwear garments and some accessories: socks, gloves, hats, etc.

WOOLEN Shorter yarns, more bulky, less twist, more warmth.

WORKSHIRT Lightweight denim or chambray, bluish colored shirt worn for work, also coordinated into casual fashion look.

WORSTED Longer, combed yarns, tightly twisted, less fuzzy, crisp appearance.

W.P.L.A. Wool Products Labeling Act. 1939 legislation stating that wool must be labeled.

Recycled/reprocessed Wool from cuttings and scraps from the manufacturer. Is returned to fibrous state and rewoven. Lesser quality.

Reused Formerly used or worn.

Virgin First use of wool. Finest quality.

WRAP Garment which overlaps part of the body. Usually secured with belt or sash.

WRINKLE RESISTANT FINISH Use of resin coating to reduce amount of wrinkle on certain fabrics.

W.W.D. *Women's Wear Daily*. Fashion newspaper, published five days a week by Fairchild Publishers in New York. With international, national, and regional fashion industry reporting.

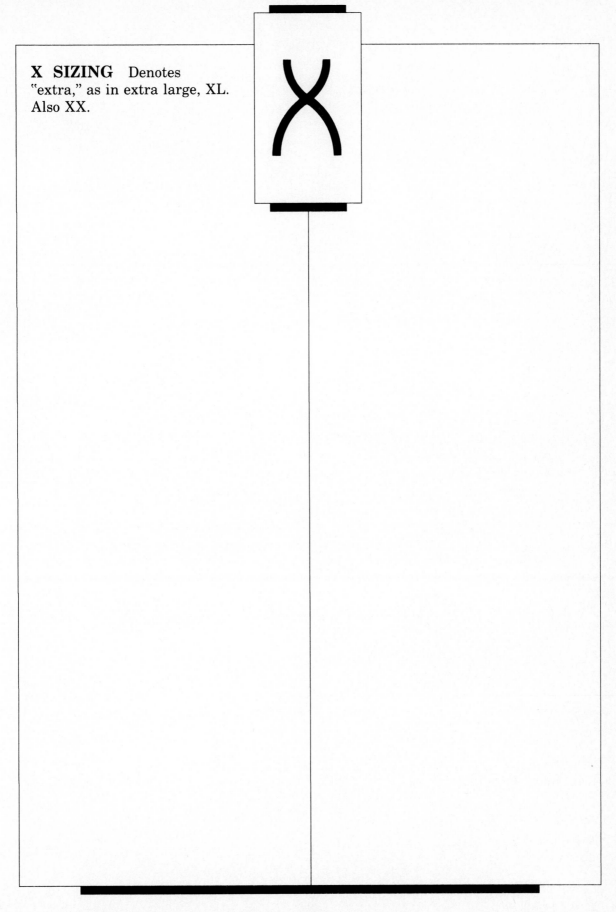

X SIZING Denotes "extra," as in extra large, XL. Also XX.

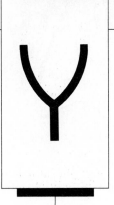

YARD United States fabric measurement of 36 inches or 3 feet.

YARN Groups of strands of natural, or man-made fibers, or fiber blends, twisted or otherwise held together, used in weaving, knitting, and other fabric construction.

YARN DYED Fibers are colored in yarn state before fabric construction begins.

YOKE Small fitted portion of garment. A separate piece, shaped with dart removal. Typically found at: 1. base of neck, upper chest, or back area. For example, blouse or shirt is attached to shoulder yoke. 2. Below waist, over upper part of lower torso. Pant or skirt is attached to hip yoke.

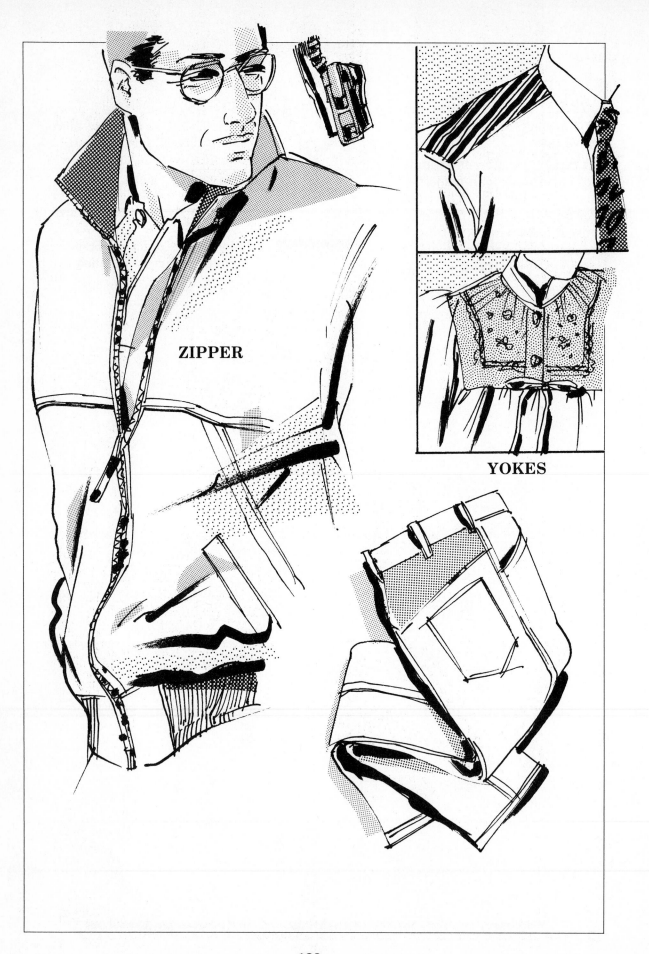

ZIPPER

YOKES

Z

ZEPEL® Finish applied to fabric for water repellency and stain resistance.

ZIPPER Closure, consisting of parallel rows of interlocking "teeth." Opens and closes by means of a tab pull. Teeth of zipper are on a fabric tape which is stitched to garment opening. May be metal teeth or lightweight nylon. Molyneaux used first zipper in high fashion in his tube jacket in the 1930's. The first zippers were bulky, tended to jam, and ran off their tracks. Oversized metal zippers have been used as design decoration. Heavier metal zippers usually used in jeans. Invisible, special type zipper—After stitching, both teeth and tape are not visible when zipper is closed.

ZIRCON *see* Gems

ZODIAC Astrological sign named for star constellations.

ZORI Straw sandal with two straps between toes and over foot. Of Japanese origin.